REHAB ALL-STAR

EXPERIENCES & ESCAPADES IN SUBSTANCE ABUSE TREATMENT CENTERS

KEITH JAJKO

ISBN: 978-1-959457-09-1 (paperback)

Published in the United States by:
Blue Jay Ink, 451 A East Ojai Ave., Ojai, California 93023

*For everyone who endured addiction to alcohol
or drugs, past, present, and future.*

TABLE OF CONTENTS

FOREWORD

Ever had one of those friends you thought would go on to do incredible things? Break down barriers? Make history? Every group of kids has one. Mine was Keith Jajko.

We first met in 1985 at a ballfield in Canoga Park, Calif., in what was at least then a bad area in west San Fernando Valley, a suburb in the City of Los Angeles. It was a Sunday night, and I was there for a softball game with my team, the Irish Creamers. He'd tagged along to watch the game with my girlfriend at the time, Diana. He was her ex. They both lived in Simi Valley, past the northwest border of the Valley in Ventura County.

My first impression of Keith was: *Jock*. Straight up. He was wearing a Beatles T-shirt (or something similar); and I was surprised there wasn't a letterman's jacket slung over his shoulder. I was wearing a band tee (sleeves cut off, of course), so he immediately started talking about music. Scorpions, Rush, Zeppelin, etc. – let's just put it politely and say I wasn't impressed with these bands. In 1985 I was three to four years deep into punk rock, and the bands that were blasting out of my little Toyota pick-up truck were Social Distortion, Black Flag, and Minor Threat. He was a nice enough guy, though.

Keith didn't play that night, but he mentioned being an infielder, and we just happened to need one. We all quickly agreed he would come the next Sunday and play, on a trial basis. So Keith shows up a week later in full-on baseball play attire. Head to toe. He might have even had eye-black grease rubbed onto his cheeks (*jock*, I told you). He had also brought one of his buddies, Mike Jacob, supposedly an outfielder with a rocket arm. Second base was where we needed a player, so that's where Keith went, which happened to be right next to me at first base. Top of the first inning, it might have even been the first batter, some dude crushes a screaming one-hop liner up the middle. Keith, with the fastest reaction I'd ever seen, three steps and a dive, snags it on a tricky short hop. Takes his time getting up, and throws a dead accurate strike to me at first and we get the guy out by five steps. I swear to God when that ball hit his glove he was on the *other side* of second base. He followed that up with a solid game not only in the field, but also at the plate, and made the team. We nicknamed him the *Human Highlight Film*.

Diana the girlfriend moved on, but Keith did not. He and his buddy MJ (the rocket arm promise was accurate) became fixtures on the team. You build kind of a bond, sharing the same side of the infield, and that certainly happened for Keith and I. As we got to know each other better, I even started dragging him down the proverbial punk rock rabbit hole. Though he'd already been getting a dose of that from MJ.

There was another thing about Keith that differed from myself. He was going to college. An actual university. That wasn't in my world at all. I was enrolled at community college but rarely attended. And I was starting to learn, through our conversations, that Keith was a very smart MF-er.

Fast forward a few years, with a different softball team, and the drinking associated with the Irish Creamers era was getting heavier. The new team was the Shindiggers, with Keith and I once again anchoring the right side of the infield. I shared a house with a few friends that we dubbed *"The City."* We had big parties after weekly games, and drank heavily (as well as some "other" things) and stayed up way too late on a work night. A usual occurrence was that when I got up in the morning, Keith would still be in the front room, face-planted into a couch or chair, the only person left from the party. It happened a lot. But I didn't think much of it, because we all partied a ton. It was the '80s and we were young, after all.

The years went on, and as I slid further downhill, Keith continued to excel. Despite our heavy partying, Keith carried on at California State University, Northridge, until he got his degree in journalism in 1990. One memory that always sticks in my mind from that period was the red Converse All-Stars high-top sneakers Keith wore, adorned with *'placemats* on the side soles of each shoe with a thick black marker in homage to his favorite band, the Replacements. A total punk rock move.

In the '90's we were still playing ball together, in Simi Valley on a team called Rotten's Row. I wasn't around as much those days, besides for softball, since I lived in Newport Beach far away in Orange County. But I was able to keep tabs on Keith's accomplishments at our after-game beer drinking sessions at the Treehouse bar. And they were impressive.

By this time he was already married, had kids, and owned a home. Right out of college he became a staff writer with the local Simi Valley newspaper, and not long after was recruited to be a reporter for one of the biggest newspapers serving the Los Angeles area. He volunteered for nonprofits, and later became a Rotary Club member and fixture on youth sports fields. He worked for an elected Ventura County Supervisor, then for a state Assembly member. All of our group's conversations about Keith revolved around the fact that we sincerely thought he'd end up being mayor one day. Maybe even governor. He was that accomplished.

By the mid-2000s, I had gotten it together a bit. I'd started my own business and moved to Las Vegas. I'd kept in contact with Keith over the years, but in 2005 I reached out with a big ask: Would he help with verbiage for my company's new website? He immediately answered *of course*, and I directed him where to find visual images of my work. What he put together, quickly, blew me away. It was dead *nuts-on*, exactly what I hoped for. More, even. The dude just had a way with words. His writing stayed on my website for over a decade.

* * *

As the years went by, I heard rumors from back home about Keith having a substantial drinking problem. I moved to Vegas, so I'd been out of touch with some of the old group, since we weren't playing ball any longer. Everyone talks shit, and Keith had always answered my calls and helped with *everything* I asked for, so I took it with a grain of salt. I even drove up to San Fernando one time, in the northeast quadrant of the Valley, on one of my many day trips to Anaheim during this century's first decade, to see him. He looked and seemed just fine. He'd seen the graphics work I recently did for the Angels baseball team – and asked for a playoff banner from the series against the Red Sox, his favorite team. I handed over the banner, we had a hug, and I was back on the road to Vegas. I saw zero signs of a drinking problem.

Fast forward to 2012. I was by this time, via my business, a main sponsor of the Punk Rock Bowling and Music festival in Las Vegas. Keith and I kept in sporadic touch to stay on top of my basic website and media writing needs, as he had continued to help me. I knew he was a huge fan of the band Rancid, who were the headliners that year at PRB, so I offered him three all-access passes, and he brought along his son and his son's buddy. They showed up at the Sam's Town bowling alley to cheer on my team as we bowled in the qualifying round of the tournament. He was clear-eyed, in great shape, and stayed 'til the end. We agreed to meet back up that evening at the festival. I arrived early, being a sponsor, and was surprised to see Keith already there, beer in hand. I didn't even think about it, because again, I had never seen signs of a drinking problem. We stayed until the end of the show – that night's closing act was NOFX. Keith seemed a little buzzed, but nothing major. My team had qualified for the finals of the bowling tourney the next morning, and Keith said he would be there for support.

So, Sunday morning we're all back at the lanes warming up. No Keith. Warm up ends and we start the game – no Keith. We win the first round to advance, move to another lane and I look around and still no Keith. We play our second-round game, lose and get eliminated, and he still hasn't shown up. Now I started to get a little worried. I called and sent text messages, no response. I headed home to change, feed my pups, and get ready to head back to the music festival.

I get there early again, as always, hoping to find Keith waiting. Nope. Call and text again, but nothing. I thought, maybe he's on his way or something. Rancid was playing that night, and no way he'd miss it. I got wrapped up with friends and acquaintances for an hour or so before I realized I hadn't seen him. Called and texted again, to no avail.

About an hour after that, I got a call. It was either from his son, or his son's friend, I can't remember. The night before, Keith had gone on a drinking binge and went missing. I was told this was a pretty regular occurrence. I was shocked. No one knew where he was.

After the festival wrapped up and I was clear of my responsibilities (this was a Tuesday) I started reaching out to some of the old gang in Simi Valley to ask about Keith and heard more stories. And about the recovery efforts that began in mid-2009, and inpatient rehabs by early 2012. And the one time that, while umpiring a youth softball game drunk, he fell and face-planted on home plate. It was all pretty unbelievable. He was the smartest guy I knew. He had consistently helped me with my business for years.

I began keeping better tabs on him. After the PRB event, he'd be in and out of rehabs, and I heard he moved down to Long Beach near Belmont Shores where I lived before moving to Nevada. In 2019 I needed him again, and same as every other time I'd reached out for help, he was sober and in good shape. I had landed the contract to do all print and install for the Raiders football club, which had just moved to Vegas from Oakland and were ready to play in a brand-new stadium. Part of my deal was getting a radio ad promoting my new contract. It needed dialogue, and once again Keith came through. Together we created a brilliant ad – and Keith even threw on a poll at the end to drive listeners online. For all the stories I kept hearing over the years, all I know is he was sober and able to help me *every single time I called*.

What I didn't know, and would learn during a wild July 2025 scramble to get Keith back on track, was my requests for his professional help were luckily timed well. The assumptions that Keith was sober all those times was a mirage. He somehow pulled off projects then. The trouble eventually was that he could no longer pull it all off. His life became completely and sadly unmanageable.

* * *

I've been around people who drank and did drugs my whole life. I was probably the biggest culprit myself back in the day. But I was always able to walk away when I'd had too much or just felt done. I've had a few friends who were not as lucky; and several are no longer with us. Keith is lucky to still be alive – because he's among the ones who could *not* walk away. And the thing about Keith was, he was really good at hiding it. I'm not trying to infer that he was hiding it from me. That would be hard. I would know; I've been around it too much. I sincerely believe that all those times through all of those years that he helped me with writing, that my timing was just fortunate.

A really hard part for me, because of the fact that I *could* walk away from it, and eventually cut out partying almost completely, was I could not understand where Keith (or my other friends) were coming from. How they were feeling, or what triggered them to throw away sobriety after such long stretches. And I regret this. I wish I could have helped more, that I could have been a better friend.

After years of communicating only electronically, I saw Keith in person in May 2023. I'd set him up again with passes for the Punk Rock Bowling festival. That year had some bands I knew he loved, especially Rancid, the Interrupters, and Bad Religion. He flew out from Maui with his friend Karen and spent the whole three days with us, at the start of the bowling tournament (it's a real thing), and at the music fest. He stayed sober the whole holiday weekend. This was the Keith I loved.

Shortly after that weekend, I called Keith with maybe the biggest ask of all. Would he help edit the book I was about to start writing? Once again he said, "*Of course.*" It took seven months of writing every day, and emailing Keith two full chapters a month. He edited as we went, sober and with me the whole way. Between the writing and editing we talked almost every day. He was sober for at least a year and a half. Then one day he dropped off. No more pictures of sitting on a beach in paradise, no more humorous social media posts – no more responding to my emails or texts. He was gone, again.

I knew his friend Karen only from PRB, but we'd connected on Facebook, so I began messaging her. He was back in the same rehab on Maui, which meant the first two weeks were restricted, no phone, no outside contact. I knew he was not fond of returning to rehab. But he did something different. He started writing a book, to use his experiences in rehabs to hopefully help others considering substance abuse treatment.

Once he was out of rehab, he went directly to a sober-living house, which I felt he preferred over inpatient rehab. Once he was into his transition, he began converting his book from ink and paper to digital documents. Upon sending me a chapter at a time, I shit my pants. Hookers, hotel rooms, drugs, guns, sleeping on the streets in winter … I won't say any more because you're about to read it. But I was in utter shock. I had no fucking idea what he'd gone through. As he emailed me chapter after chapter I was in disbelief. You readers have no idea what you're in for here. Buckle up tight.

* * *

He was writing everything in a manner that was similar to the way I wrote my book. He wrote about different times and eras as he went, often out of order, with the intent of making chronological sense later. Only he never got there. I never got the last chapters. Keith once again flew off the tracks and went missing.

He surfaced at the emergency room in the local hospital, which I had learned by now was a pretty usual occurrence. People find him on the streets and call 911. Karen set it up so I could speak with him on the phone there. He was shit-faced drunk when I finally got him on the line. It was the first time I'd ever talked to him when he was in that shape. And it was *bad*. This wasn't the Keith I knew.

From there he returned to the same rehab, under the same rules of no outside communication at the beginning except for written letters (which could be inspected, or so I learned reading his draft book chapters). I wrote him a couple of letters and sent a copy of my book, which by that point was published. I learned the date of his discharge and looked forward to talking with sober Keith again. At the time of this latest relapse, he had rented a small apartment and was not living at the sober house. When he was released from the rehab, he went directly back to the apartment (instead of to a sober living program for the crucially needed *after care*) and relapsed soon thereafter. I never even got a chance to talk to him before he initiated Blocked-Up mode.

I want to talk for a minute about the title of the book: *Rehab All-Star.* When I first heard it, I thought what most people probably think: he's been to rehab so many times he's considered an all-star now. But, no, Keith's too smart for that. What he actually meant is that *while he's inside the rehabs and sober living houses he's an all-star.* Because he thrives there. He's sober, goes back to being super-smart Keith, and actually helps run the places. He uses past job skills to help with the administration, with marketing or communications, and property literature and procedures. He offers advice in areas to help stay compliant with regulations. He literally is a rehab all-star.

* * *

By July of this year, I realized I needed to do something. This dude had helped me *SO* much through the years. I felt a need to help him get back on track. Through Karen, I set up a four-day visit. With her as the middleman, Keith agreed to sober up for my time there. It didn't happen. When they picked me up out front of the Maui airport before noon that sunny morning, Keith was shit-faced. He'd already drank an entire pint of vodka. It was super easy to find the car with Keith slur-screaming out the passenger window. When I got in the car I could smell him – like he hadn't showered or changed clothes for days. Karen suggested we go to lunch somewhere near the beach, which surprised me. I didn't think they would let Keith in. When we arrived and exited the car, it was worse than I thought. He could barely walk and had huge open scabs on elbows and knees from falling. He was wearing flip-flops and one of his toes was torn up so bad it looked like it was about to fall off. Karen bandaged him up right there in the parking lot and we went inside.

We kept him sober most of the day. They drove me around showing me the sights, and by the end of the day Keith had sobered up and was talking semi-normal. He had asked several times, somewhat forcefully, for a beer while we dined, but I shut him down. At one point late in the day we were trying to walk to some cliff where divers jumped into the ocean. There was supposed to be a lot of divers off the huge black rock at sunset every night, but Keith couldn't make it. We walked only about a hundred yards, and he said he couldn't go on. However, when we arrived back at the apartment after dark, Keith immediately exited the car and said he was walking to the store to get booze. He'd tried to get Karen to stop on the way back to the pad. I asked her how far he had to go, and she said about a mile down a hill, and then a mile back up to home. And it was a big fucking hill. But he did it. He couldn't walk a hundred yards down a beautiful beach on a gorgeous day in paradise, but he could do almost a half-marathon to get alcohol.

When he returned, he was huffing and puffing and had already guzzled a third of the pint. Then he sat down at the same back yard patio table with us, and I watched him drink another third, directly from the bottle. I was trying to talk him into stopping; and finally I think Karen and I talked some sense into him. He poured out the last of the bottle and the plan was for her to babysit him until he went to sleep, and then we'd work on getting him to rehab in the morning.

I slept in an upstairs spare room and woke super early to try to catch him before he woke up. When I got downstairs it was 6 a.m. or so, and he was rummaging around his apartment. He'd forgotten pouring out the last of that pint and was looking for it. And again, even though I was pleading with him not to, he once again ran the gauntlet down the big hill and back for vodka. So, Karen and I sat there and watched him at the table in the backyard drinking vodka straight out of a pint bottle. It wasn't 7 a.m. yet.

I started on him again (with Karen's help) about needing rehab. He said he dreaded the idea of rehab again, preferring instead the sober house. However, that wasn't how it worked. He'd need detox and clean-up before the sober-living house would allow him in. He kept mentioning this guy Chopper.

I made phone calls before the trip reaching out to some of the old gang, some of Keith's longest friends, and asked if I could call while on Maui, so they could let Keith know how important he was to them and that they were cheering for him. Almost all agreed. With fortunate timing, our friend Mike Jacob called right when the bottle was half empty, and I'd almost convinced KJ to dump the rest. We talked on speaker phone for about 10 minutes, then MJ told Keith he loved him, and we disconnected. Keith immediately started crying. I then talked him into dumping the rest of the bottle.

All through the morning Keith kept talking about this Chopper guy and the sober living house. He was wasted, and not making much sense, but I could tell he respected the program. So Karen and I hatched a plan: let's talk with Chopper and see if he'll consider taking Keith directly in, instead of requiring rehab first.

Chopper managed the sober-living house in a program Keith had been in and out of pretty much since arriving on Maui at the end of May 2020. At one point he'd lived there for three consecutive years. It was still morning when we arrived, in a town called Kahului not far from the airport and beaches. And there was a really nice Harley-Davidson chopper parked right smack in front of the residence. I knocked on the front door, and after a few minutes a tall skinny guy walked out and looked at us. He said, "*Aw, man ... Keith*" with a sadness in his voice. I guessed it was based on Keith's appearance and obvious state of intoxication. I introduced myself as a lifelong friend from the mainland to help him get better. I gave him some background and asked if he'd consider taking Keith back in without a rehab stay. This is exactly what he said: "*Of course I will. We love Keith.*"

Chopper asked for some time to get paperwork together, and get a bed arranged. We took Keith to breakfast, and to a drugstore for some medication and gauze for his wounds. When it was time to return him to the sober living house, I began worrying about this part. See, in the draft chapters of his book, there was a long passage about this exact part of the process. Once again, I had a stroke of super good timing, and the pre-arranged call came in from our longtime friend Mark Benner. I put him on speaker and explained exactly what we were doing, and Benner, an old-time punker like us, offered some extremely heart-felt words. Again, after the call, Keith cried. He was definitely feeling the love.

We were minutes out from Chopper's – the hardest part. I saw Keith gazing out the window and knew what he was thinking. From the back seat I said, "*The Ride to Rehab.*" From the passage from his book. I guess it settled him down, and we arrived with Chopper outside waiting for us.

We all went inside, and Chopper showed Keith his new living area. Super clean and spacious. He explained that Keith would be on "lockdown" for two weeks, with routine pee tests, which Keith readily agreed to. I could see it in Keith's eyes – he was already feeling at home. I gave Keith a big hug, told him I loved him, and would talk to him as soon as he completed lock-down (and got a new phone, I learned later, because he loses everything in relapses). I turned around and was given a big hug by Chopper, which I wasn't expecting. I could tell he sincerely cared about Keith.

And that's where I left him. Last time I saw him. I called Hawaiian Airlines to change my flight home to that afternoon. Two days earlier than expected. I'm super stoked to report that as of this writing, Keith is thriving at Chopper's. He's already completed and formatted his book, and is deep into editing and fact-checking. He's helping Chopper best he can to keep the house in top shape. Keith is once again being a Rehab All-Star. A difference now is, he's firm on the importance of remaining grateful, and actually utilizing tools and tactics to one day be an all-star away from rehab, too. Hopefully, his days as a *real-life Little Leaguer* are past.

James Swanson - August 2025

PROLOGUE

"Imperfects are used to indicate ongoing or repeated past action."
Merriam-Webster dictionary

Summarized, *Imperfect can represent a past action in progress but not completed.* So it seems I'm an imperfect.

My story is rather atypical for alcoholics and addicts. If there is such a thing as typical as it relates to human beings with imperfect brains.

By my early 30s, I'd enjoyed significant successes, perhaps more so than many at that age. I won awards in my professional field, was honored by employers, served boards of directors for nonprofit organizations, assumed community leadership roles, spent two years as president of my college journalism alumni association board, bought homes, married a wonderful woman who raised three children, coached more youth sports teams than I can count, traveled some, made plenty of money, and more. But it all teetered on a dark secret which for many years remained confidential. For quite a long time I kept an unhealthy consumption of alcohol and drugs – part of my life since high school – hidden.

Not many people who consume as much as I did can keep the secret for life. Most are simply discovered, their problem spotted by friends or family members (who too often don't let the sufferer forget). More of them – or should I say us, meaning addicts, which includes alcoholics since *alcohol is a drug* – just lose the ability to handle it physically or mentally, or both. It's not that anyone discovered the severity of my dilemma; the problem became too enormous to hide. It took a while, but when it was time to take my life away, my addiction obliged. I'm among a great percentage of addicts who reached a point where the body no longer could process the poisons. From that point, my body and brain would malfunction in some fashion, sometimes moderately, most times absurdly, whenever alcohol or mind-altering substances were ingested, smoked, or injected.

My body couldn't break down the toxins fast enough, or sufficiently, putting a considerable amount of pressure on my brain to manage. Like the proverbial bucket being overfilled, such situations drowned and overwhelmed and made a mess. People who reach the same point – which can be triggered by *anything*, like money woes, work situations, or problems with the law – could right the ship and avoid the poisons for good. A significant percentage of sufferers might relapse, maybe more than once, but ultimately they attain the relief and freedom of long-term recovery.

I am not among them. Recovery didn't "catch on from day one," as they might say in recovery meetings. I didn't go to one rehab and stay free of toxins happily thereafter, like some rehab colleagues. I've had numerous relapses, continuing to the point of this writing. My lapses in sobriety are persistent, like a bad wound that won't heal. I have recurring, *unrelenting* relapses, which always seem to get worse any way you measure them. Hellishly bad.

While I've had a few notable periods of sobriety, even surpassing a year in length, and once reaching 23 months, I uncontrollably veer to the old fall-back of alcohol. These relapses precede an awakening, akin to miraculously surviving through a terrible ocean storm, where, as it subsides you feel as if alone on an island oasis ready for another chance at life. These oases were substance abuse treatment programs, commonly called rehabilitation centers, or rehabs. The number of rehabs I experienced is embarrassing to admit sometimes. Like it or not, it's my major thrust for this book: **to help others avoid what I did.** The intent is to share memories from each rehab facility and provide not just anecdotal observations, but real-life examples of *what life can be like in rehabs*. Some details are difficult to share, but I try to be as honest as possible because those particulars could help someone.

I started writing this book while in one of my last rehab stays. As I wrote by hand, around the midpoint of my six-week program, a newcomer in his first rehab said in a group, "I knew I needed rehab, but I was scared."

It reinforced why I was writing out memories of the five rehab facilities I experienced, plus some experiences in between. People avoid rehab because they don't know what to expect, and it's unfortunate. How many are injured or actually die because they fought off the need for rehab treatment? (See my chapter on the year 2017 for insight into the dangers of this phenomenon).

I hope to help ease anxiety about inpatient treatment. Rehabs are not complicated; yet they are not entirely unchallenging. Most anyone can enter and complete rehab regardless of socioeconomic standing, race, gender, religion, or any other way we're identified today. There may be a wait depending on availability of open beds, or maybe challenges with proximity if no beds open nearby, but with diligence and persistence anyone can try.

Rehabs are mostly the same; yet, not the same. There are common denominators, which I try to outline. Yet each has its own approach for getting people clean and sober and (hopefully) keeping them that way. That last part is vital. I can easily *get* sober. I just stop drinking or doing drugs. What I struggle with is *long-term maintenance*, which is more difficult (and time-consuming) than stopping. Sure, stopping drinking or drugging is difficult, often very much so. But quitting can be initiated immediately and achieved in a brief period of time. Stopping can be accomplished by sleeping a few days without ingesting poisons. *Remaining* clean and sober, on the other hand, needs ongoing attention daily.

Put it this way. Imagine being diagnosed with glaucoma, if the results of an Intraocular Pressure (IOP) Measurement exceed a certain level (in my case the number 24). With a little time using medication eye drops nightly, that number could decline noticeably, and other tests may not reveal anything alarming. An eye specialist at that point may be inclined to discuss it rather nonchalantly, something like, "The numbers look good … It looks like the drops are working." Yet, *ongoing treatment is crucial for managing the disease and preventing vision loss.* What the ophthalmologist should have added is, *"Be absolutely sure to continue using the drops every night."* Or even also, "...

because if you don't, you could go blind within years."

It relates to treating alcoholism or addiction, and at least I can acknowledge it today. I'm no expert on recovering from alcohol abuse disorder, substance abuse, or addiction. More than a dozen rehab stays over a 15-year period proves it. I'm not qualified to help individuals get sober and stay that way. What I *am* experienced with is excelling *while inside rehabs.* I don't know if that's good or bad, so the following is a deep exploration into the subject based purely on experiences and observations. My hope is to avoid editorializing or sermoning too much, and skip the temptation to overly analyze studies, statistics, medical jargon, or various approaches to addressing addiction legislatively or politically. I simply lay out real rehab experiences and associated emotions, and let readers choose what to think or how to proceed. Kind of an old-school journalism approach: let individuals read and react, as they see fit individualistically.

Hopefully along the way readers can gain a nugget of knowledge (or two or more) to help with decisions. Such choices can be among the biggest a person can make in a lifetime. That is, whether to go for it, and accept help, and combat the mind malady of addiction once and for all.

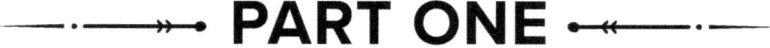

PART ONE

INTRODUCTION

STORY OF ANA

I hadn't seen her in years. In fact I wouldn't have recognized her had she not called out my name, inside a crowded hallway inside my eighth rehab stay for treatment for abuse of alcohol and drugs. Let's call her Ana, and she looked terrible. Fellow drinkers recognize signs of a rough spell: anything marring the facial area. Bruises mean drinking was likely involved. Cuts bigger than shave nicks mean most certainly alcohol contributed. Ana had one and all: remnants of a black eye on one side; and on the cheek opposite more than one scratch, plus swelling. A potpourri of facial flaws, if you will. Alcoholic stuff.

All sorts of memories surfaced. I remember how it had taken Ana years to find her man, but once she did, you could sense the man ended up with a very caring wife. I can't remember how many times I heard about her step-son and his exploits in active duty, I believe with the Army, or maybe Marines. Whichever, it was in the Middle East and he was there a long time. Ana mentioned him every time we spoke over many years. Strangely enough, she ended up marrying a law enforcement officer. I say strangely because when we were younger and hanging out, we usually made the cops chase us around town all night. We were no angels, for sure.

At this rehab – it was my second stay there in the San Fernando Valley operation, the first being five years prior – Ana shared sad news. After so many years of marriage to the man it took so long to find, Ana's husband died suddenly. I didn't ask how; I assumed it had something to do with the heart or health considering the occupation and stress. It was irrelevant. My first thoughts were, My Lord, how will she get past this, from a recovery perspective? Talk about being dealt a tough hand. I lost both parents a few years apart during my long recovery journey, but that's hard to compare with losing a spouse suddenly and unexpectedly. Any death of family or friends is perilous for those in recovery. Ana had surrendered her whole life to the man, and she seemed content, and I admired her much for that.

By this time, in August 2018, I don't know how deeply involved she was with recovery, but I knew she had at least some experience with what can be referred to as *our world*. I'm confident she did at least one rehab stay before I began my tours of them, which was 2012. I remember after completing my first rehab, we connected by phone and, while I cleaned my garage sober, shouldering the phone to an ear, she lectured on all sorts of recovery shit. Stuff I'd just heard in rehab, so it seemed familiar. I did a lot of mm-hmms and uh-huhs as I swept. It seemed weird talking about recovery with an old friend. That's how green I was at the time. My brain still had remnants of what I'll call the Hiding Mode. Early on, it can be typical to keep thinking you're not an alcoholic or addict, so why jeopardize friendships or relationships by letting on that you have a problem? Most alcoholics and addicts start recovery by believing things will return to "normal," whatever that is. Today I accept that I am abnormal due to faulty brain wiring, and talk freely about addiction or recovery with anyone who asks. I don't seek it or push it, but I'm less hesitant to openly share what I know.

The reason is, you never know who you might help, or even save, with a single sentence. I know the 12-step programs are big on maintaining anonymity, and I understand. You can be damaged by letting on that you're an alcoholic or troubled by drugs. It could prevent you from being hired, and the employer probably won't divulge the reason. On the job, it could result in harassment or worse, like working without potential for advancement. You can be secretly exiled. Any of those reasons could trigger relapse.

Which may be why those early talks about recovery with Ana seemed uncomfortable. I agreed that I had a problem *at that moment*. By that time I'd been attending AA meetings for three years, and during that period appreciated the directive that we should hide our fellowship membership, as an anonymous participant. The only people who knew about my recovery efforts that began in mid-2009 were my wife, parents, and doctors. My kids may have had an inkling. Plus, all the strangers in AA.

They weren't always strangers. All kinds of people I already knew walked into AA meetings in our hometown of Simi Valley, Calif. While considered a big city by federal standards, Simi in fact was sort of insulated by mountains surrounding it, and for some reason felt smaller than the reality of about 125,000 residents. In AA, I would see opponents from political campaigns past (which for me explained much, haha); old high school buddies (who might call out your last name when they first see you, busting that anonymity thing all to hell); or people I worked with professionally over the years. Pretty consistently I saw familiar faces in that room off Tapo Street behind McDonald's.

People like Ana. So I wondered if she had a foundation solid enough to get past this terrible personal loss, without experiencing the horrific extended relapses that us serious alcoholics endure. The older we get, the more painful the relapses, a reason for my concern for my friend while standing in that hallway, both of us starting our 50s decade in age.

When I asked what brought her there, her response was unsurprising. She drank, she drove, she crashed, and here she was, a veteran rehabber joining another. I relayed my story about a harrowing escape from a frightening sober living house in Compton, Calif., and by luck landing there at Tarzana Treatment Center days prior. I explained that a relative of a high school classmate worked magic to get me a TTC bed immediately, skipping the typical waiting period that they always seemed to say is around 60 days. So I had this free rehab ride without an end date, which I felt was needed. I was in bad shape.

Being back at TTC reminded me of my first stay there in 2013. After about four months, I escaped out a side door to the waiting car of a girlfriend. It felt like a jail-break operation in the dark. The then-director of the entire program, a bona fide asshole, had turned the place into a detention camp. I was done with it.

This is an example of rehab bullshit one may encounter at any treatment facility. By that time, deep into my fourth rehab stay and first at TTC, I achieved the point of obtaining passes to visit the library or government workforce development office, to access computers to look for employment that I would need to save money to rent a place to live after rehab. I was homeless when I entered, and the plan was to follow what everyone else seemed to be doing: get in a sober living house, to continue what is called *after care.*

I never made it. Director Asshole initiated the odyssey by announcing one night – through his assistant of course, since Director Asshole couldn't be bothered communicating directly with us lowly clients – that the entire "house" was closed for a week. That is, no privileges, like getting passes to leave campus and seek employment. The house closure would last until everyone snitched out everyone with drugs on the property. Director Asshole was convinced someone was slinging dope inside, which I agree cannot be tolerated. You can't have that stuff floating around in a treatment environment. Not only could it take multiple people out (of the program that is, via relapse), but it could have fatal consequences. Addicts away from their drug for an extended period have their tolerance to the drug diminish. Should they suddenly return to the drug, a tendency is to use the same amount as before, a volume they last remembered using. With the tolerance reduced due to abstinence, addicts have died from this judgement error.

I understood the reasoning for the shutdown. It was unfortunate, but not the end of the world. But when not a single person stepped forward (surprise!), a week later in an all-house meeting, Asshole's assistant announced another week of closure. The culprit this time was mobile phones. They knew we had them, and until we turned them all in or snitched everybody out, the lockdown continued. This one moved me some, since I had an iPhone stashed in my room. How else would I follow baseball's World Series? Addict young adults there dominated our recreation room television and never allowed sports or anything else on the tube. So I sweated it out. I lived in a dorm with six bunk beds, housing 11 or 12 dudes at a time. Someone in there could have seen me with the phone. Also possible was that someone might want passes reinstated. Snitching on someone could get the lockdown lifted. So I laid low.

So did everyone else, and staff collected not a single mobile phone. So, back to another all-house meeting we went, expecting the lockdown to end. No client had left campus for two weeks and some of us were getting annoyed. But, alas, the assistant program director once again apologized for the bad news, but we'd have another week of lockdown. This time they expected couples to step up and turn themselves in; or snitches to out secret couplings. Most rehabs that allow cohabitation of the genders have strong rules against over-fraternization. It makes sense, since attaining long-term recovery is very difficult, and requires tremendous attention and dedication. How can you focus on recovery when the mind is preoccupied with another person? Relationships are one of the two top reasons for relapse; the other being failure to get the help you need (per a counselor years later in Hawaii).

I understood the staff's concerns with the couples there, and indeed there were plenty, but I was pissed. I didn't have an end date to get out, but I'd already been there over three months and felt it was just time. My counselor was little help with arrangements for post-treatment care, and in fact would not guess or divulge when I was supposed to be done. It felt like the song "Hotel California." I could check out, but I could never leave.

So that first TTC stay ended with a rush under darkness to the car of a girlfriend, who had just secured her own studio apartment in our hometown following the failure of her marriage. This person, by the way, also was in and out of recovery, so it ended up being a fateful decision. It's a bad idea for two people both early in recovery to attempt a relationship. One goes out, meaning resuming drinking or using, and the partner usually follows. In rehabber parlance, it's called *taking out* someone. I told friends more than once, "She took me out." (When in reality I let myself be taken out).

The problem there was, in that relationship, half the couple *never got into* recovery. We arrived home that night and on the kitchen table was a bottle of wine and a bong. I lasted about a month sober while she drank and smoked, even walking a considerable distance to AA meetings, but eventually got the proverbial haircut and joined her. Hang out long enough at a barbershop, the saying goes, and eventually you get a haircut. Moving there ended up causing a significant amount of pain over many months. It was a dark age. Live and learn.

* * *

Back at TTC at the start of Stay No. 2, Ana explained that her insurer approved only 14 days there. Without hesitation in my mind I thought, *not enough.* For an alcoholic of Ana's caliber, two weeks of treatment is hardly worthwhile. It's basically an extended detox. What very serious alcoholics need the most is *time*, meaning, time away from the substances. They need to get that time any way possible. Extended stays in residential rehab helps.

Ana needed 90 days at least, per my uneducated and untrained opinion. Probably more. But I never expressed that to her, and regret it. In our hallway, meal time approached and we separated. Due to rules already mentioned, Ana and I never did get to talk further. Last I saw her was on a visitation day, walking down the hallway with her parents, who knew me. In fact, Ana pointed me out and her parents waved. For a spell, I was darn near part of the family.

But after that, Ana was gone. That rehab was weird with exits. I don't recall many of the typical graduation-like ceremonies common at other rehabs. At TTC, people either got kicked out, which most of us either witnessed or heard about; or they simply disappeared. I took the latter as kind of a joke, as in, "Hey, where did Joe go?" Or, "How peculiar, we haven't seen Joan in a while." *Twilight Zone* stuff.

A few months after last seeing Ana, I was ejected myself, for sneaking out on a pass although it had been revoked. It was canceled because dumbass kids in our dorm of 14 people were still in bed as breakfast time approached. Without phones, and few watches, we kind of relied on each other to get everyone up and going for the day, so we could all make our beds like good little boys and leave our living space nice and tidy. But that Sunday, young dudes kept sleeping, and none of us noticed. Until a program assistant (PA) who looked like a yard duty Nazi straight out of the movie "Porky's" came waltzing in and began yelling. She went berserk over the sleepers, and we knew it would mean trouble once regular staff came in the following day which was a Monday. And it did, hence losing my pass.

Well, as with the first stay, my mind was stuck on the belief that the most important thing in my life was working to make money, which meant spending as much time as possible on a computer applying for jobs. So that morning, I left the property anyway, heading for a place to donate plasma for money. I must have hit a liquor store on the way back, because I woke up the next morning in an emergency room bed somewhere not far away. Apparently I'd returned to TTC blackout drunk, and they gathered some of my stuff to carry with me in the ambulance to the ER. The next day I went back to TTC to get the rest of my stuff, because the beginnings of a hand-written novel were there, but after being ignored in the lobby for about an hour, I gave up. Fuck it, less to carry, was my thought. That's how the alcoholic mind works. *Fuck it* is not just a saying; it's a feeling, a state of mind that should be avoided at all costs. Getting too much of the *FIs* will take you out.

Immediately, life got rough. I survived a harsh spell of homelessness bouncing between Simi Valley and Long Beach, Calif., which are not near each other freeway-wise, and I had no car. I learned to bus-train-bus long distances. Eventually I meandered home to Simi Valley, with plans to spend Christmas with my father, who was still reeling from the passing of Mom in 2016. It's an understatement to say Dad was displeased to see me at his front door, but he let me stay. We developed a plan where I would stay there a week or so until a bed opened at the rehab I'd graduated from earlier that same year. The year 2018 that seemed to never end. So through Christmas and the days after, I sobered and enjoyed spending time with Dad. During this period he insisted on driving me to AA meetings, so I wouldn't be tempted walking by all the liquor stores en route. Good call, Dad.

We had great talks on the short drives up and down Tapo Street. He cared and asked questions about AA; and I tried to answer best I could. Best were the return drives when I could offer a play-by-play of what just happened in a meeting, like a sportscaster, only keeping out names. Mostly. Once, the kid of an old friend of mine, who Dad coached in baseball long ago, was in a meeting. I told Dad, and after a later meeting he had a chance to see his former player. (My friend's kid, by the way, was sadly taken by his addiction a few years later).

One day near the end of 2018, via a social media app, I received a message from a woman I did not know. She was a friend of Ana's, and had an important message. That month, Ana relapsed, the friend explained. As anyone who is or has been a heavy drinker knows, one does not simply stop alcohol after an extended period of hard daily drinking, without medical attention. You get sick, called detoxing, and sometimes terribly so. On several occasions, I asked friends or my parents to watch over me in those first hours and days of not drinking, as the body slowly eliminates the poison and brain sort of recalibrates. Many times, I would have them feed me two or three beers spread out over a day or days, to taper off. These were not easy decisions for people hosting, but I was persistent. Stopping suddenly, e.g. cold turkey, for a very heavy drinker is dangerous. I know; I had a seizure in June 2016 on the second day of trying to recover right after re-entering the Salvation Army. It cost me days in a hospital bed with a constant Ativan drip. The experience is about the most frightening of my drinking career, and that's saying something, all things considered.

Ana's friend wrote that our friend passed away. Very shocked, I asked for details. The messenger said Ana relapsed, then while stopping she detoxed badly, and suffered a seizure while standing. She fell backward and smashed her head hard on the ground, causing her death. Shocked is an understatement. I felt I'd just seen her, smiling with her parents in that rehab hallway. Honestly, I didn't know how to react. I didn't tell my Dad, nor anyone in AA. What I did do was stay sober long enough for Dad to drag me off to Long Beach for another rehab try. Rehab stay No. 9 would commence at the beginning of 2019.

While I felt a desire to reach out to Ana's parents, I never did. I didn't tell Dad, nor friends who knew Ana, or anyone in AA. My nerves about yet another rehab stay overpowered my thoughts at the time. It's not easy knowing in advance your intake date for rehab. It seems better to just have someone on a moment's notice take you away and drop you off.

I know this because by this time I was a Rehab All-Star. I kick ass inside rehabs. I get elected to patient leadership bodies, take on major responsibilities, sometimes more than one, and rarely break rules (well at least serious ones) or lose my temper. I am very rarely late to anything. I get along with staff, almost all the time; and group sessions inside classrooms are not bad. In college I learned to sleep with my eyes open – a key skill in programs with schedules packed with classroom-like sessions focused much on un-sexy subjects like behavioral therapy.

While I might be an All-Star on the inside, out *in the real world I'm a Little Leaguer.* I am not someone who can consistently apply everything learned in treatment programs, on a daily basis as needed. I constantly require "refresher" courses, revisits to rehabs. Essentially I became a rehab crasher. I crashed rehabs like I used to crash back yard keg parties in my youthful heyday. One among thousands of us in America who keep trying for that Holy Grail of permanent sobriety.

In fact, from my third rehab stay and thereafter, I encountered other rehab crashers I met from previous rehab stays. Like discovering a former

TTC detox roommate at the Salvation Army a couple years later. "Repeat customers" are common. A reason is that recovery is fucking hard. Not to bore with statistics, but let's say out of 10 people in any given rehab class, one might make it. Sometimes, maybe two of 10. Meaning, maintained sobriety.

This is a story about some of my fellow Rehab All-Stars, and some crashers, and our experiences, good or bad. I try to supplement information with background into what has grown into a multi-billion-dollar industry: substance abuse treatment services.

This book is for parents or friends of sufferers, or for individuals themselves, seeking or desiring help, for whom rehab is an unknown. It's to help alleviate fears about entering rehab for the first time. I know those fears are real. Remember that 40-year-old first-timer saying during a group session in Rehab No. 12, that *he was scared about the thoughts of rehab*? I didn't bother asking what he was afraid of. I knew. Lack of knowledge about what's in a rehab, not knowing how hard or easy it will be, uncertainty about how long you'll have to stay. Not knowing what it will be like afterward, should the program get completed and full-time sobriety begins.

Not knowing what life will be like without alcohol or drugs ever again.

This tome is also for myself, to help in my continued recovery from my diagnosed, life-threatening mental maladies. That work, maintaining sobriety, never ends. Let your guard down for a day, or even for just a moment, and Hell can return where it left off. This is no exaggeration. To summarize, I hope the following words help someone out there who could use a little dose of hope.

* * *

Some notes on names, and sober living houses. First, laws are strict about maintaining privacy for health care patients, including for those in rehabs. So most names in this book are not real. There are a few exceptions. A handful of friends approved use of their names, and I chose first names only for a less formal read. This is not a journalistic report nor a study-driven textbook. It's a memoir about a single (albeit major) element of my life. A vast majority of names here are pseudonyms.

Secondly, while some sober living houses and experiences are mentioned, this book does not come close to properly offering my experiences in these "transitional living" or "halfway" houses. This book focuses on experiences in regulated rehabs. I consider sober living houses separate from true rehabs. Sober living houses are more on the side of after-care recovery maintenance, and are not government-monitored (except maybe by local land zoning regulations, for things like overcrowding or zoning violations). A sequel focusing on the sober living house world may follow, but this book is about rehabs, with a few segments about periods between rehabs. At times I felt it important to outline what I did (and did not do) between rehabs.

CHAPTER 1

BIO ECONO

Tour-Spiel

The chapter title is from a saying by the Minutemen, a 1980s punk rock band, describing how they could musically kick ass, but economically. They would *jam econo* – without electronic enhancements, musical wizardry, concert pyrotechnics, laser shows, or "funny stuff." What you saw was what you got. The Minutemen would just plug two guitars into amplifiers, next to a modest drum kit, and let it rip.

In that vein, I don't see a need for minute detail about my life pre-treatment and -recovery. Let's just say I was an over-achiever who squeezed a lot out of ordinary talents. I gathered skills and attained success in a number of areas of life, all by a relatively young age. I offer the following to set the stage for the storms outlined in the chapters to follow.

Basically, I did what was expected at the time for a middle-class white kid from the suburbs. Born of parents who worked long hours for the postal service and regional telephone company, I behaved best I could. I had good grades in school, made plenty of friends, never got into fist fights (away from baseball fields, that is), and lettered in sports including baseball where teammates my senior year elected me team captain. I dabbled in trouble but consciously avoided what might hurt others. Me and my troublemaker associates were at least a little socially conscious that way. I tapped kegs well at backyard parties – earning the nickname Keg Man from some fans – and got to chat with police officers more than most of my peers. I was carefully daring, I guess you could say. A rebel without a clue.

I went to college, which took longer than usual because I had to work jobs throughout, and eventually attained that bachelor's degree. It was my family's first college degree, both sides. I won a $10 bet with my grandma

Char by graduating a semester before her, in her quest for a bachelor's degree after teaching at a private Catholic school for a quarter-century. I graduated in May 1990. In the middle of college, a significant change blossomed. I discovered punk rock music, and a new world and attitude that came with it. I always had a rebellious side, but punk made it feel more purposeful, more disrupting, more *free of care*.

I majored in journalism, and was a rarity going right to work in the specific field of my major. I became a staff writer for my local daily newspaper, where I did well enough for 18 months to get recruited by a much larger competitor, a major metropolitan daily newspaper in Los Angeles. As hard as I found the work – and indeed it was very challenging – I just kept pushing forward and excelling. I was young and had little real world experience, or even much knowledge about communities or institutions. I learned fast and became the proverbial jack of all trades. The utility player on a baseball team, someone who could play any position at any time. It's quite valuable in a career, I learned.

I wrote hundreds of articles over four years in newspapers, probably over a thousand in total. I learned to report and write on any subject as ordered, and had creativity to develop story ideas where others saw none. I was curious, moderately skeptical, and noticed little things around town. I often just wrote about what I saw. I won a couple of minor local press club awards, one for a piece on the emergence of a local alternative rock music scene, another for a deep look into why high school sports programs in my hometown seemed to dominate that period. I was, and remain, a storyteller. I grew to love the little community I called home, and most of my work covering Ventura County reflected it. One year, I had more bylines than any other staff writer at the *Los Angeles Daily News*, something like 400 articles in 365 days. In mid-1992 I married a sweetheart midwestern transplant, Lisa, and two years later we welcomed our first child, a son named in honor of my childhood hero, baseball legend Hank Aaron. Lisa and Aaron live in Ozark,

Missouri today.

I met many community leaders, among them a city council member who won election to a higher office with the county. Unlike the city council, the county gig came with paid staff. She recruited me mainly to manage the media, and help with writing and other office demands. With all the experience and contacts from reporting, I excelled again. I loved that job. I spent the last half of the 1990s getting paid to help people in my community. I learned a heck of a lot about how the government works, and how to deal with unpredictable people. We also had two more children, both daughters, a year apart almost to the day. Co-workers were amazed that it seemed Lisa was always pregnant, or we were celebrating a newborn. Haha. Katie and Maddie made our family of five complete.

I also kept getting asked to serve on the board of directors for local nonprofit organizations, starting with the Boys & Girls Club of Simi Valley, where I was vice president of marketing the entire time I worked for the county. Over a period of about 17 years, I served the board of directors for a Rotary club, the local Friends of the Library, the Free Clinic of Simi Valley, the Moorpark College Foundation, a university alumni association, and a girls softball league. I was president of the Journalism Alumni Association at my old university for a couple of years; and at one point served as president of the girls softball league board.

I got shit done. Due to this, I was consistently asked to do more.

I also bought a condominium, then sold it to move our growing family into a four-bedroom single-story house where we lived for 13 years. The home was nicely located two houses down from my parents and the house where I grew up. I was just grooving in life. I achieved a dream and coached kids on the diamond, my son in baseball, the daughters in softball. And I kept playing adult recreational slowpitch softball through my 30s. I attended rock concerts regularly, goofed off consistently, and was not exactly "growing up." I felt destined to always be a 17-year-old trapped inside an aging dude's body.

All along, I consumed too much booze and knew it. It never seemed to get better, or the amounts smaller. They say once you become a pickle you can never be a cucumber again. As hard as I tried to cut back, or craft my addiction into some acceptable form, I never came close. The path always went one direction, the wrong way. Yet I persevered relatively unscathed.

The trouble was not sudden. The mass consumption of beer began mid-high school and never subsided (until I first tried recovery about a quarter-century later, in mid-2009). Deep into my professional career, I peppered cocaine into party sessions. Sometimes I'd snort lines off my desk at work if alone. Early in my career I tried LSD and ecstasy (MDMA), and I smoked pot now and then when it was around. However, cocaine was a constant all the way into the new century. Almost anyone who worked with me in the 1990s had no idea. Perhaps due to my personality and the jobs involved, most everyone assumed I was just a hard-charging writer and drinker, a Hemingway-like character. That perception may have helped me get away with hangovers, looking rough in the office, or calling in sick for work – sometimes for days at a time.

Despite the unsteadiness of the substance use, my professional career wouldn't slow down. In 2000, I was hired by the then-largest public relations firm in the nation, representing large corporations from an office in downtown Los Angeles. The experience was exciting, at least at first, being just 33 years old with only a journalism degree, swimming with the sharks in a big-business and hyper-political office in the city. However the commute proved too time-consuming considering three young children at home. I burned out fast.

I made a lateral career move, taking a job managing communications for a national trade association in Chatsworth, maybe a 20-minute drive from home. What a relief it was to drop the tediously long commute. They loved me at the association. I was honored and praised by management, and just flat-out excelled managing up to 14 people in four departments. Yet, fate intervened. Or, should I say, greed. The *attraction of more* overwhelmed my sensibilities.

While with the association, a land-use development firm planning a new-home master plan in Moorpark needed public relations help, and called to ask whether I consulted. Having just learned with the PR firm how to work by contract, I knew about the billing process. I wrote a contract for $1,500 a month, and they accepted immediately, paying me while I continued working a full-time mid-management job. Hooray for the advent of email and mobile phones. The money overall was almost unbelievable for this guy with shaky confidence about his management skills, who never took a business class. This dude living with an enormous lie, abusing alcohol and cocaine secretly. It felt like, as they say in AA, faking it to make it.

Later I was offered a part-time job directing communications for a friend who was an elected member of the California Assembly, the smaller house of the state Legislature. His party tabbed him as minority whip, a position that brought additional funding for his office, which he used to hire me. For just 21 hours a week, the position paid well, and came with impressive state benefits which was important with a family. With the new job and the consulting gig, I quit a stable, full-time job with great potential for upward mobility, meaning I was on track to becoming an executive eventually. It was a fateful choice, not just for my career, but for my mental health.

* * *

At the time, many longtime friends from school were cracking six figures in salary, becoming executives, and buying big houses in fancy neighborhoods. The economy thrived due to the nascent tech industry. Additionally, there was a huge housing boom inflated artificially by new bank loans where anyone could get cash to buy property, regardless of credit worthiness. It was boom times, and I didn't want to miss out on bounty just waiting to be claimed. That's how it felt.

I worked 20 months for the Assemblyman, until his term was ending so the party replaced him as minority whip. By that time, however, my land use consulting contract had grown to $5,000 a month, no taxes removed.

The latter part would be painful once I didn't have taxes pulled from my state check. Internal Revenue Service woes are significant, and stress causes more drinking, and also makes it hard to stop. True story: more than once, I included the IRS in my AA Fourth Step list of people or institutions for which I held resentments.

Within a month of the layoff, out of the blue and unsolicited, a tech company focused on internet banking for mid-sized financial institutions called offering a part-time position managing communications internally for its 1,700 clients nationwide. It was the last months of 2004. What was explained as part-time work ended up being nearly full-time, as I was paid hourly and was on-call if any product outages occurred, or if a product update was planned, which was constant. Much of my work was dictated by contracts with banks; we were obligated to communicate quickly for anything unusual with product performance.

I became a digital spreadsheet and mass emailing expert. I'd be called at 1 a.m. to email 500 banks affected by some problem. They provided me with a laptop with a special new virtual private network gizmo, so I could safely log in and clock in any time from anywhere. I made a tremendous amount of money for work that was rather technical but not too difficult, for a company making so much money that no one questioned my hours. I just kept getting asked to log on, and kept getting paid. They even made me an official employee, so I got benefits including paid time off for vacations (which we did for a week at a resort on the west Maui coast, capped by a helicopter ride around the island). In the big book of Alcoholics Anonymous this would be called playing the Big Shot. I most certainly was.

In a two-year period my income surpassed six figures, by quite a bit. It felt like we couldn't spend money fast enough. We were young, easily afforded the mortgage, and liked to have fun. With the freedom of working from home, I coached youth ball teams, and still played fairly high-level slowpitch softball at least once a week. I served the governing board for the Moorpark Rotary

Club, and began doing marketing projects for small businesses. I took it all as if it all was routine, that it would last forever. We did not save nor plan for any rainy day. There definitely were signals that troubled waters lay ahead. What I didn't know is that, for me, that Moorpark housing development and its income would end up creating a Stage 5 hurricane personally.

I was first arrested for driving under the influence at age 19, in 1986. This was just months after crashing and wrecking my first car, a 1966 Ford Mustang bestowed to me by its only owner, my grandfather. I'd been drinking before the crash, but police never arrived thanks to the very friendly driver of the other car, and a fast-acting father who drove me to the hospital and somehow arranged for the Mustang to be towed from the scene. The classic car was totaled, and I spent summer months riding a bike to a hospital for work before getting another vehicle.

I had other contacts with police, but nothing major. Still, though, deep into the 1990s I was doing an awful lot of cocaine, and drinking and driving too much. In my professions – first as a news reporter with random drug tests, the other as a political aide who could make headlines with an arrest – always in the back of my mind was it all could end fast. That bothered me for a long time; I was conscientious of an evident problem. It did not, however, deter or even slow my consumption of poisons.

The second DUI came in December 2002, at the end of my stint with the trade association and before work with the Assemblyman. I literally was awaiting the offer from the lawmaker's office when I was arrested. I would have understood if they backed out, but they took me on regardless. Luckily my reputation for writing and media and political work was solid. I'm still grateful they did not back out; it was a wonderful experience.

Around this time, cocaine started becoming harder to find. My main provider found love and exited the business, and by that time I was too old to have connections. I couldn't find it on my own and wasn't about to try. It's something to note here that I never really *chased* drugs (at least not until

I moved to Long Beach, in 2015). In fact, I rarely paid for any. Drugs were just available, or provided by who I happened to be with. Eventually I would look back and realize that I was a true addict, that while alcohol is my drug of choice, through the years I was addicted to cocaine also. Years later, I would spend a whole year, 2017, addicted to crystal methamphetamine. If drugs are readily available, and I'm drinking hard, or in a state of vulnerability, I'll consume drugs like I used to gulp beer by the gallon.

By 2005, I was replacing cocaine with the legally available liquor. Three things happened over a period of about five years that changed my life, without exaggeration. First, in spring 2006, voters in Moorpark rejected the housing project that paid me handsomely since 2001. What could have been a decade's worth of a nice monthly retainer, as they built out the project, disappeared in one night. Poof, and $5,000 a month evaporated. I was lucky that the county supervisor I formerly worked with took me back on a part-time basis, as she needed assistance with her re-election efforts, but it lasted only to the end of 2006. We lost the re-election; it was a terrible year for me and elections.

Luckily, one of her close friends, a leader in town, connected me with a national home-builder who was having a contentious time with neighbors of a project they were trying to build in south-central Simi. Besides a monthly contract just to be the local communications contact for that project, the company offered a matching contract to also be the public relations specialist for its entire North Los Angeles division. I wasn't making $140,000 a year any longer, but it sure didn't take long to gain back $5K in income. I was making more than most people I knew, and my wife still didn't have to work and stayed home to raise kids well. It was a wonderful setup for the family that I look back on with fondness. I'm very grateful that I didn't lose time with the kids due to commutes or demanding corporate office work.

However, immediately after I took the new contract gig, at the very end of 2006, the economy crashed hard. It was like Great Depression-level bad. The worst part was, the industry most impacted was what brought most of my income. Home sales crashed with hurried new loan regulations. Records would be set consistently for foreclosures, and this went on for several years. It caused record numbers of layoffs, and business closures. It worsened and lasted at least half a decade.

Each year my contracts were halved, or disappeared. A $5,000 monthly contract became $2,500, then just a year later, cut back to $1,500. Retainers went away. I started to scrape to bill hours for pay. Land use developers might bring you on for a project or task, but either they let you go once the task was completed, or they would get cold feet and drop you with little or no notice. It became very difficult to run a business. For a long spell I felt always on edge; I couldn't stop thinking about how to generate more income. Plus, it's really hard to find and land new gigs when your brain is blocked up most of the time from booze. A tipping point neared.

I kept coaching youth baseball and softball teams, joined a local free clinic board of directors, and somehow kept landing just enough work to keep our family train rolling. However, unpaid taxes would haunt us, and the stress of hustling to bill hours while constantly looking for new work took a terrible toll on this human psyche. I first turned to wine, for more of a punch-per-glass than beer. It was what older, established people drank, after all. My excuse was I was *maturing* (Haha!). The switch to wine was the second big development of the trifecta that ultimately took me out. Quitting the promising full-time job in 2002 set the stage, but losing the big 2006 election and switching to more potent alcohol fanned the flames.

When the wife noticed me drinking too much wine out of big plastic cups designed for soda or beer, she commanded no more drinking in front of the kids. That's why wine was among the big decisions that eventually combined to wipe me out. Wine built up an already high tolerance for alcohol, because I drank it in volumes equivalent to my beer guzzling. From the moment of my wife's stern order, I had to keep drinking, but now also had to hide it. So I turned to vodka. Smaller bottles, easier to hide, a smell more easily covered. Vodka changed me from a successful young professional with executive potential, to the depths of Hell that I struggle with to this day.

It was Strike 3, but I still didn't sense big trouble. In my mind, eventually things would improve with the career and finances, because *it always worked out*. I took my luck for granted. I underestimated how badly my brain and body were declining due to stress and poisons.

The beginning of the end occurred in late April 2009, when I collapsed in a public setting and the shit really hit the fan.

Perfect Storm

At the end of April 2009, I was umpiring a girls fastpitch softball game before hundreds of parents in a game between top teams of 8-year-olds. In the second inning, I collapsed, first forward onto my face mask right there in the batter's box, then, upon getting back to my feet, backward until I stumbled all the way back into the wood backstop. I hit my head hard somewhere along the way.

Fans, confused at what they witnessed, initially believed I suffered a diabetic reaction. The game was halted, and I was dragged to a small table behind the backstop, where my finger was poked for insulin levels, while we waited for an ambulance. My friend John, on the league board of directors with me at the time, was not fooled. Not long into the game break, he said quietly to someone we both knew, *"Get him out of here!"* John took my truck keys while another friend drove me to the hospital, skipping the ambulance ride. John later delivered my truck home.

At the emergency room, my blood-alcohol content was 0.34%, a stunning level of toxicity, but nowhere close to my recorded high (0.44% a few years later in Barstow; I had a streak around early 2013 of cracking 0.40% regularly). Note that half a percent of alcohol in your blood, or 0.50%, brings stupor, and possibly death. Longtime hardcore alcoholics are aware of the 50 magic number. I was ingesting much more alcohol than I assumed, yet remained hardly concerned. Doctors and nurses sounded the alarm, but the numbers didn't register with me. Yet. The hospital didn't keep me long, and I spent the night at my parents' house because my wife was out of town, my son was home under my care, and no one wanted me to sleep the night due to a suspected concussion. It was a touch-and-go evening.

The following days were difficult. The first morning and day, I discovered what I kind of knew: *I have a lot of good, caring friends.* Word spread quickly, and many called. The next day I spent a lot of time crying while talking on the phone. I was scared. Humiliated, certainly. Mystified, and perplexed about what was coming. No possibility that I could drink freely again, to norms I spent years establishing. What I'd used to feel good and ease anxiety for a quarter-century was now a threat to my life. On top of that was dealing with the damage to my reputation, especially with the league, of which I served as president just the year before and remained in a new past president position. I was greatly involved with youth sports for several years, and hundreds of parents knew me.

I had a good family practitioner to see, and I will never forget the session the next morning. Besides expressing some shock – I was perceived as this no-nonsense working professional – and conveying the seriousness of the situation, my physician advised that I had *a lot of work* to come. In the end, she held the sides of my face with both hands, pulled me forward, and looked closely straight into my eyes. I can't remember the exact words, but the memory is chilling. Essentially it was, "You poor soul. You have such a long road ahead." Maybe she added something like, "You're going to need God." I don't remember. I was in ultra-shocked mode.

There is not a doctor alive without experience with the eternally frustrating alcoholic, or as modern vocabularists would say, a *person with alcohol use disorder*. A huge percentage of visits with physicians involve alcohol consumption, either due to a mishap while intoxicated, or a health ailment caused by extended use or abuse of the liquid drug. Abuse of ethyl alcohol is a life-threatening illness with no cure. In other words, a doctor's nightmare.

Of those who attempt sobriety, no more than a fraction attain it and keep it. Some say the number is about 5% to 10%. Could be a little more, but in my experience, not by much. Certainly no more than 15%. I always assume that one in 10 make it. You can sit in a room of 20 AA members, hear them speak, and think how miraculous the program seems to work. A newcomer may ask, *Look at all these people sober! And … happy!* What new visitors should know is, among that group, only one or two will maintain recovery. The rest will at some point relapse, and many will not return. It's a strange phenomenon to witness if you stay involved with an AA group over an extended period. People disappear. I often wondered, *Where do they go? How peculiar.* Besides the one or two lucky souls among a group of 20, the rest move away, stop coming altogether, die, go to jail or prison, or live on miserably somehow. The latter tend to not live to ripe old ages. Alcohol damages so many organs and bodily functions; the list is long.

My doctor pulled strings and got me in with one of her college class-mates, an addiction specialist physician *and* psychiatrist who was not taking new clients. I was lucky to get in the next day with my doc's urgent reference. He happened to have an office not far from my physician's. I didn't like him. Of course I didn't: his job was to tell me I couldn't drink. He was friendly enough, even had a decent sense of humor (which is important in recovery, by the way), and I appreciated the effort to try to help. I just felt … so helpless, and so very tired. I was almost too exhausted to listen, absorb, and digest information properly. My innermost self knew I needed help, but my thinking brain just couldn't accept it. It was hard to swallow that I would need pills the rest of my life. I was only 43; and could never again drink alcohol freely.

Prescribed for me was what he termed a *triangular program*, involving medication, group therapy, and individual therapy. Many years later, this very formula would provide my longest period of sobriety as an adult, from August 2021 to July 2023. However, that would be years away. In 2009, I could have accepted and executed the triangular program, and today I might have 15 years of sober and clean time. That physician-psychiatrist specialist was spot-on from the start. Too bad it wouldn't be until around 2018 that I stuck with the meds. Once I began adhering to the triangular program, as managed by an intensive outpatient program eventually, things seemed easier. I wasted a lot of time by not listening or acting as directed by medical professionals.

My recovery journey began in mid-2009. I attended dozens of AA meetings, and met with the addiction doc regularly, first every other week, then monthly, and eventually every other month. I didn't know it at the time but what he had me on was an outpatient treatment, or OP. It's kind of like being in a rehab, only without having to live inside a facility. Years later my insurer provided what is called an *intensive outpatient program*, or IOP, where you not only see a doc, but you're pee-tested weekly, and attend classes three days a week for many weeks until it is cut to once a week for ongoing maintenance. It is indeed, intensive, at least at the start.

While connected with the OP doc and his program near my hometown, I stayed sober for about a year. I had faith in the medications, at times giving them credit for my clean time, belittling how much AA was helping, or even the doc or my therapist. I found a private counselor who I liked and saw consistently. Just talking candidly an hour every week or so, one-on-one, seemed to help. She was unassuming and super friendly, in a small office with candles, dim lighting, and a chill vibe. She talked directly, straight at me, relaxed and with sincerity. She was good at remembering my crazy thoughts and details to that point. I bought into it. I'm a kid from the late 1960s and '70s after all; the hippie-Zen stuff doesn't bother me. Overall, I did the deal, as they say. I understood it all decently enough; and deep in my innermost self felt it a little of the spiritual stuff so many around me seemed to mention. I felt pretty darn good, for many months, cruising.

Which is not the best place to maintain sobriety. You don't cruise. You work hard, and fight like hell to keep what you have. There came the day, which happened to be Memorial Day weekend 2010, about a full year into sobriety. I was under meds and had the cute therapist and Doc Mohammad and AA and such. I had it going on. Then, that first drink came calling. I sipped three beers that Saturday with some younger high school classmates. I noticed they drank, but didn't do what I would, which is continue drinking one at a time until I needed help. But my lizard brain had inscribed into my memory a lasting perception of pleasure; a memory of what in the past succeeded in releasing dopamine. What made me feel good.

It can be thought of this way. The brain and how it developed over 40 million or so years, is how it is due to *experiences*. The reason we're alive is, our brains have very carefully developed ways to avoid danger, and also to feel good consistently (which I see as a trick for us to exercise, or at least remember to have a little fun). So we would not be eaten by tigers or killed by really big things or by accident. Something like that.

A lesson was learned with this first relapse: when with friends, if *they know I cannot drink*, I don't get urges. I've attended class reunions bone sober and don't remember being tempted. But around friends who *didn't know?* All bets were off. It's a weird phenomenon. I knew this, but it helped me little. I just remember how easier it felt when friends really close to me knew that I should not drink. They were never vocal about it, but for some reason I behaved.

Those three beers initiated a slow, long period of hiding drinks, pushing it to where my intake volumes increased steadily over many months. I experimented with everything, like low-alcohol beers, even high-cost imported fake beers. I discovered BevMo in town and its great selection of fake suds. I dabbled with pre-mixed club soda-based drinks in small cans, which might taste like a margarita, or vodka and tonic, or something. Mostly they taste like shit. The main thing was they packed a punch, and the cans were small and easy to both hide and dispose of. The ability to transport, hide, and dispose of alcohol containers is a big deal for those who abuse alcohol, I learned.

Most friends believed I was sober through 2011, but it's untrue. The wife began to notice, especially as the year wore on, whether or not she'd say much about it. She was actually nearing the end of the line. Yet she stayed, and for a long time put up with it. For work, somehow I kept one large client, to bring in at least some income. And (*finally*, in my troubled mind) the wife began working full-time for the local school district. It helped a little financially, and a lot for health care coverage. Eventually, she said she stayed because she loved me. That she believed in me and my fighting spirit, which she predicted would win the day. She used to say, "Just go for the W," referring to *the win*. I liked it, but ... my condition was way beyond inspirational slogans.

She didn't know, as most "normies" don't, that a human being's individual spirit or strengths are *useless against addiction*. Loners might attain a temporary reprieve. However, for darn near every addict, the reprieve is brief. To last, it must be supplemented and nurtured by a lot of work and love. Actually it's a lot of work, hopefully daily, involving people close to you and even folks you don't yet know. To summarize: going it alone is a recipe for failure. Don't try to get sober alone, or let an addict try it. It's a damn hard lesson to learn. Right away, once you have a problem that requires assistance, you have to humble yourself to others, often total strangers. It's just how it is. When confronted about the trouble for the first time, the lizard brain can take over, and then comes the lying. Here's the conclusion many of us make early in terms of being *stuck in rehab*: This is temporary; play good and get "paroled" as soon as possible; then fake it, somehow, maybe forever. Yeah, that's the ticket.

That slow-developing relapse lasted from May 2010 to early 2012. Roughly 22 months of a snowball growing in Hell. It took someone who dearly loves me, my wife, to take action and save a life. The era of outpatient treatment was over by the end of a dark February 2012. No longer could I chase fantasies of past successes, and just do anything I wanted as long as I generated income. It was the proverbial turning point. I graduated. To inpatient rehabs.

CHAPTER 2

ABOVE IT ALL
LAKE ARROWHEAD, CALIF., 2012

Lifehouse

At the end of February 2012, I reached my end. The wife, armed with excellent health insurance from her school office job, researched and found a rehab with an opening. A *residential* rehab, that is. A real one, where I would live, and not be home or with anyone I knew. She talked me into it, amazingly, and I vaguely remember relief in accepting. With little warning, as fast as her pretty soul would move, she had me pack a single bag of clothes and toiletries. Then she drove us about 90 minutes away, far off, and up into the mountains of Greater Los Angeles. She made a good call not wasting time from the moment of *discovering a rehab opening*, to *transporting the addict*. This is a key, very brief period of time. Looking back, the lack of advance notice was a good thing. I struggle to explain the hodge-podge of emotions that kick in during drives to rehab. Be forewarned: it's rough.

I did not know this during the drive up to Lake Arrowhead (plus, I was at least a little intoxicated), so this first ride was unremarkable. Still, my first suggestion for those considering inpatient treatment, whether for yourself or for another, is to free the vehicle from all anger, resentment, or any other negative thoughts. Keep the vibe optimistic, as positive as you can pull off. Mainly I mean for the driver, or whoever else is in the vehicle with the transportee. An addict can go insane on a ride to a rehab. Know this. Don't assume they won't jump out of the car and run away at any opportunity, like on a restroom stop at a gas station, or on the freeway in a moving car. I am not making this up.

I know quite a few words, and usually can explain subjects with decent clarity. Still, I cannot adequately describe the emotions involved with transport to a rehab. Confusion, anger, resentment, sadness, frustration, more anger, anxiety for sure, some terror even, hopefully some empathy for loved ones you hurt and left behind. Fear of the unknown, or even fear of the known if it's returning to a rehab already attended. I know the rides to rehab stays Nos. 2 and 3, to the same location and operation, were *way* worse mentally. I knew ahead of time what was coming and there was no way out of it. I felt like Dead Man Riding in those cars. Removed from society, maybe never to be seen again. At that point, delivery people, you might as well allow a drink or two during the drive. It could help, in my opinion. In terms of the addict's situation, it pretty much doesn't matter by then. A little alcohol in moderation could help ease anxiety and more easily get them to where they need to be. I admit to sneaking an airplane bottle shot of vodka while the wife drove me to rehab stay No. 2. I feigned the need for a nap, crawled over seats to the very rear where I couldn't be seen, and wiggled free a tiny bottle hidden in a pocket. Slammed it and crawled forward back to the front passenger seat, as if this was all normal.

A rehab returnee will dread the memory of all the group time sitting in classrooms, or being around strangers all the time, the rules, the rules enforcers, whatever. When you know, you know. Then there is the experience of *rarely having alone time*. Always surrounded by addicts, under all the rules, chores, missing your mobile phone and friends. The feeling of living under a microscope daily can get to you. Rehab revisitors know that coming soon is lecturing, righteousness, sadness for friends missed, limited freedom to make decisions (like running away). The bubbling of a wide range of emotions. The list goes on.

Sit in a car for an hour on the way to inpatient rehab and you'll probably experience every human emotion. Each visit can *seem* worse, by the way, a reason for the main theme of this book: **Get it right the first time.** Don't become a Rehab All-Star or treatment crasher. You don't have to, you don't need to, and you don't want to be a return customer.

Keep rehab delivery ride vibes positive. Crack a joke or two. My Dad, who drove me to stay No. 3 up that same mountain, said while on the trek, "Treat it like a summer camp. Think of it as an adventure!" I laughed and thought, just another dad joke. Then I thought more deeply about it, and relaxed for a better ride. I'd been there already, and knew nothing would *hurt.* No one will hurt you in rehab, except maybe your counselor taming your ego. I just came to the solemn conclusion that I needed a month's break from the poisons. Entering, I knew it was temporary. Not all rehabbers get that. Many addicts protest immediately, firmly, sometimes fiercely. Rehab is a mental test. Some manage it; others let *feelings* of threat or control by others drive a desire to flee.

* * *

In my last year of high school a teacher said write a letter to the principal, whatever you want to say, without, he said clearly, fear of repercussions. That's all I needed to hear. I wrote an essay titled, "Young rebels against old bastards." No name on the one-page screed, I felt safe to submit. Free speech, right? Wrong. They identified my handwriting, and off to the King's office I went. Confronted, I admitted my writing. I was proud of quoting Bob Dylan (even though I think I had the wrong artist), and saying I felt like a number there. I don't remember much of the discussion with Mr. Ellis, but I do know that for decades I saved the single sheet of lined paper, and always remember his brief message. He wrote, "Hey Keith (which showed impressive respect I must admit, personal attention), Abe Lincoln once said, 'A man feels how he chooses to feel.'" That's all. I never felt like I could live down the rebels vs. oldtimers vibe, especially since I wrote it spelled *rebells*. Without a clue.

The point here is, *attitude* is huge. It's vital in getting through rehab, and maintaining sobriety. Expend a lot of energy on negativity and you basically multiply how long being in rehab *feels*. You might end up feeling like you did double the 30 days you actually endured. Please, going into rehab, readers or those reading who are helping another, emphasize messages like,

"Have patience," "Listen more, talk less," "Be grateful," and, "You gotta want it." My father once put it as this. Dad and I are fans of the Boston Red Sox baseball team. Historically we hate the New York Yankees. Dad grew up in Massachusetts, anchored by The Hub, Boston. He was trying to inspire me, as he tried a hundred times before games. He said, "Pretend your drinking is the Yankees. And you want to beat the Yankees how badly?" With all my might and energy, I thought. Great idea, A for effort, but still not enough.

Avoid letting the addict beat themselves up, and *do not lecture* or harshly criticize. Your addict loved one chose to take the great leap and get into the car *to seek help.* That deserves hugs, not scorn. Remember the immediate goal: *keep 'em in the car.* The entire route, to the end. That whole project of delivering the addict to the place of help is crucial. It's almost a spiritual journey, both for deliverer and deliveree. In the end, you feel delivered away from some really bad shit.

It can take an act of God to get an addict to agree to that first rehab stay. Many of the afflicted never will. Some die first. *Get the addict in that car, or on that airplane, and you may have saved a life.* The afflicted may be unaware, but those who get them to rehabs are *fucking angels.* Not everyone suffering from the illness gets the opportunity. Some have no family or friends, or are not familiar with potential assistance from the government or charity organizations like nonprofits or churches. Those who receive help should be grateful, and then some.

* * *

I woke to the voice and sight of a huge human being named Rick. He was a counselor then at Above It All Treatment Center, a fairly high-end program where we all lived in cabins spread among the mountain woods about 80 miles northeast of Los Angeles. White vans kept clients connected to an administrative Center with a classroom, on a road appropriately called Rim of the World. We were way up high in the mountains, overlooking the vast San Gabriel Valley.

I awakened on a couch, out in an open upstairs loft area near rooms full of beds hosting alcoholics and addicts. It was the program's detox center, which was so full, I was on a holding couch awaiting a real bed in a room. When I arrived the night before, after a lengthy intake process that involves a lot of paperwork followed by searches of your person and your bag, this is where they plopped me. This big two-story house would be home for a few days.

Rick tapped me on a knee and said, "Hey, what's up, brother? You feelin' all right?" Seeing my dazed and confused eyes, he added in a comforting voice, "You're in the right place." All rehabbers will probably hear that phrase. Rick was an exceptional counselor (and still is, though somewhere else).

The place was a detoxification center, of which AIA had two. This was the main one, larger with a big kitchen, professional cook, and huge living room with plenty of soft couches. Detox is considered separate from what they call residential treatment – the true "rehab." If they say you're to do 30 days, understand that usually detox time, which is at least several days, might not count against the 30. You could end up doing 36 days total, for instance. Detoxes are hospital-like settings, with nurses monitoring, and doctor visits now and then. Except for rare outbursts, detox centers are quiet. You sleep and eat and sleep and eat. Repeat. Interrupted by nurses waking you for meds or to check vitals. I can't remember if I smoked cigarettes at AIA detoxes. I certainly did in all other detox centers.

Detoxing after a significant run drinking or drugging can be dangerous. I had a seizure in June 2016, because I suddenly stopped drinking liquor. Only alcohol and benzodiazepines, or benzos, can kill you while detoxing. People recovering from opiates or cocaine or other drugs may suffer greatly for many days, but misery is all they get. Heroin addicts who stop won't suddenly die. They'll just wish they would.

Detox nurses have to know much about each type of substance, and let's always remember that alcohol is a drug. Each substance makes victims feel differently upon stopping. There really is no detox protocol for crystal methamphetamine, a powerful drug that now commonly causes addiction. A doctor told me years later to detox off meth, all I could do was sleep for three days, and drink a lot of fluids. He offered no other protocols, not a single med. Just advice: sleep it off.

Other drugs have medications known to help soften the landing, so to speak. Ativan (lorazepan) once was common for alcoholics – for my seizure I had an Ativan drip for days. It's a benzo, and stopping that drug cold turkey, even after just a brief period of intake, causes its own bodily response. I returned to my program after the seizure and was quite nauseous for days. It took me a while to realize I was coming down off Ativan. Says artificial intelligence now, "Long-term use of benzodiazepines like Ativan is generally discouraged due to the risk of dependence and withdrawal." Alternatives might be hydroxyzine or gabapentin. There are many other non-benzo options, none of which in my experience are as effective as Ativan against anxiety and nausea.

Opiate users might get methadone, but not as much nowadays, as it has one of the longest detox periods, up to 28 days. Staying a full month in a detox center, which might have a television and some books but little else, seems brutal. In recent years, detoxes and rehabs might dispense Suboxone, a combination of buprenorphine and naloxone used in treating opiate addiction. Opiate users command a lot of rehab nursing attention, in my experience. They're just miserable, usually in bodily pain, lethargic, and almost always annoying at least for the first days.

For the rest, it's pretty much mild sedatives and vitamins. What I quickly learned at my first rehab was, *America had a really serious opioid problem*. It was 2012, the middle of the Obama years, and this rehab accepted clients of all ages from nationwide, predominantly patients in their 20s or early 30s. That first stay in AIA, I'd guess the breakdown of primary drug per resident was 60% opiates; 25% meth; 10% alcohol; and one old dude on pot. This first stay, the latter was an old stoner from Maine. When I returned in the fall just months later, it seemed the opiate problem had worsened.

The breakdown then had to be about 70% opiates, 20% meth, and three or four of us old guys who drank too much. It's rare to see someone in rehab for addiction to pot. We did one time have a guy who couldn't stop inhaling from aerosol cans.

Eventually I crawled off the couch and down some stairs to the big, open, high-ceiling living room area, where they were about to serve a chef-prepared breakfast. This place had a guy who cooked breakfast and dinner for detox patients, and lunch for residential clients served at the Center, every day. These were damn good meals. I've yet to come across a rehab that didn't stuff you with big meals daily, plus an almost endless supply of snacks. We need the nutrients after ignoring diets for weeks on end. It's like the military: An army marches on its stomach. Rehabs know addicts will use any excuse to walk out. *Their first job is to keep us there as long as possible*, not just for business, but *because it's best for recovery*. As much time clean as we can possibly get out of it. The last thing they'll allow is for someone to leave because they're hungry. New rehabbers, don't worry about meals. You'll eat a lot, and mostly it will be tasty and fulfilling. Sometimes they let you nap afterward.

A doctor will decide how long you stay. Some programs try to kick you to residential in a few days. In my later rehabs I pushed back to get more days. I'm a terrible alcoholic, and older so my body recovers more slowly. Still detoxing while sitting through group therapy sessions, as they do in residential, is miserable. If you still don't feel well, tell them. Maybe even insist on not going to residential for a day or so more. In more recent years, I was in a program where you had to walk up an outdoor staircase for meals. I knew my gait was too wobbly to navigate the stairs after just four days, and said so. They let me stay longer in detox, I think to a full week due to timing with a holiday. Some won't move you to residential on weekends or holidays.

I've done lengthy detox stays, at least 10 days, maybe even up to 14. Sometimes I think it's just a matter of demand, whether that particular detox is full, and if there's a waiting list (which most often there is). Sometimes though you hit the slot just right and no one's there. My next-to-last rehab, I spent several days as the *only* patient in detox. They shrugged their shoulders when I protested moving over too soon. They didn't need a bed at that time. That's a big strategic operation with rehabs: keeping beds full, but sometimes keeping one or two open if they have agreements with a hospital or other organization. They might agree with a local hospital to always have a detox bed open, for that "return customer" the hospital is tired of seeing.

That's commonly how they word going to residential, "moving over." There really is this physical move of locations, from a hospital setting with nurses, to rooms and hallways packed with free and wandering alcoholics and addicts. I had a little anxiety every time I was moved to residential. It's just fear of the unknown – even for someone who really knows. Don't sweat it, you're not alone having trepidation about moving into residential. All told, *being in residential is better than being in detox.* Detox is mind-numbingly boring. But it sure can be heavenly sleeping early on.

* * *

At AIA, the move over wasn't as simple as gathering your clothes and being escorted to another part of the same property. My first rehab housed clients in cabins, all spread apart, each with four to six, or even more, beds. They had a van fleet to connect us with the Center, with outside 12-step meetings, for recreational excursions, and for other transports such as to medical appointments. At every rehab, you quickly get an idea about the daily schedule. At AIA, it meant getting up, eating in your cabin, and waiting for a van for transport to group sessions.

They assigned me to a special cabin designated mainly for older, mature dudes. (They had one or two cabins just for females; and no co-ed houses much to our dismay). Our little two-bedroom cabin did not have a house manager living with us, because we were tethered by a short trail through the woods with a much bigger house, where they packed in younger clients and had a manager living there all the time. For us, it was a cushy setup. Four mature, no-nonsense fuckers with a TV, packed fridge, and hardlined phone to use whenever. I remember every morning watching "Married with Children" reruns with a trucker from Washington state who could never sleep late due to his profession. I'm pretty sure I've seen every Al Bundy episode.

We really didn't have much, besides two beds per room upstairs, then a tiny bathroom with a shower, small living room, and equally small kitchen downstairs. I think there was a wooden deck outside the kitchen but there was no furniture and we hardly used it except maybe for privacy when on the phone. It was March, so nights there were quite cold. Walking that little trail at night to visit the other house for meds or to mingle or play bumper pool could be mighty dark and spooky. I was no longer in a protected suburb. I was out in the wild, literally.

A standout element at this rehab was how they filled your refrigerator every week. I mentioned earlier how the cook prepared breakfast and dinner for detox, and lunch at the Center for residential clients. In the mornings and evenings, we in residential were on our own to prepare our meals. Each cabin had a refrigerator, and each week we would fill out this order form indicating what we needed. These forms had everything from steaks, cases of yogurt, who knows what else. Sometimes forms changed. Regardless of our supplies, we ordered more each week, so much in fact that they had to start stacking breads, dry goods, and fruits on top of our kitchen table. We couldn't eat it all fast enough, and they never said anything about the hoarding. The kitchen table was usually almost completely covered, forcing us to eat meals sitting on a couch or reclining chair in the living room. Bachelor stuff.

Luckily, our truck driver housemate was a good cook and liked to do it. Sometimes he'd treat us to a full-on breakfast plate, but more often he did chef-quality dinner meals. When I arrived the fridge was absolutely packed with things I loved to snack on, like cases of yogurt. Every week I'd order another case. And, maybe some ice cream, or ice pops. We were amused by the system. These cardboard pallets of yogurt were stacked four-high at the bottom of the fridge. The freezer was looking good, filled with ice pops and ice cream. Sometimes we'd experiment with the form by checking something exotic that they listed for whatever reason, just to see what would happen. Most often, lo and behold, it would be in our kitchen when we returned Wednesday afternoon. Looking back, it was surreal. We had a barbecue out front, too, which we didn't get around to using. But we sure as shit ate well. No one was going home skinny.

As with almost all my rehab stays, the big item each day was the schedule and class-like meetings called *group* sessions. Every weekday morning there was like this check-in group in the spacious living room at the big house down the trail, where we'd all talk and share for an hour before the vans arrived. Sometimes we had the first group right there in our cabin or our big brother one next door, so we stayed. Other days, we'd pile into vans and go wherever the groups were hosted, most often in the big main room upstairs at the Center.

The Center had offices downstairs for administration, and these volunteer counselors we'd meet with so they could accumulate hours required to become a certificated counselor. I don't know what differentiated them from the main counselors, which each of us were assigned to, and who in reality were in charge of our individual recovery programs. There were four main counselors, and for my first stay I happened to get the chief counselor, in charge of them all.

My first counselor was excellent. I remember not deep into my stay, maybe two weeks in, I happened to get the shotgun seat next to him in a van as he drove us down the mountain to something in San Bernardino, probably a 12-step meeting. Without any prompt from me he asked, "Keith, have you ever thought about a career as a substance abuse counselor?" I responded pretty quickly with what I would probably still say today: No, I couldn't deal with *everything counselors have to handle.* All the people, and all their personalities, problems, and, especially, the fibbing and trying to game the rules. It was true then, and I still feel this way. I couldn't stay sober if I did their job. No way. On top of it all, the job didn't pay very well, which is unfortunate. Have respect and empathy for these counselors. They're angels, too.

Which brings us to my next recommendation, about staffers. Addicts quickly learn what detox is, compared with residential treatment, and who are the *bossy people*. Those can be counselors, of course, and sometimes detox nurses, but more often it will be folks there to assist, commonly called *program assistants*, or PAs. Most are pretty cool and helpful. Others are assholes who need new careers. Most addicts don't like being told what to do, always a challenge for rehab staff. Well, the job of a PA is to tell us what to do. Instant conflict.

So, you have detox where a nurse will always check your vitals and give you happy pills and make sure you eat. You're pampered. Some are better than others but every addiction rehabilitation center has one (except the Salvation Army's Adult Rehabilitation Center, to be explained later). You can't take someone in active addiction, or shortly out of using, and stick them in a dorm and, especially, classroom seats. They'd get pissed, disturbed, maybe even ill, which only promotes the desire to flee. Remember, a primary goal of rehabs for very early recovery is to *keep the client there*. Keep them in program, to get time under their belts, and wait for the magic.

Ending an addiction to a mind-altering substance begins medically. It did for me in 2009 with the outpatient services of an addiction-specialist physician and psychiatrist. It did every other time I escaped a big relapse, except for the Salvation Army. Stopping the ingestion of powerful toxins is no joke. Besides having the potential to kill, if the halting is not handled well it can reduce the chances of success. Very early on with addicts, it can be quite touch-and-go. It is imperative to *keep the odds for success as high as possible*.

Attaining sobriety, and keeping it, is very hard. It's the most difficult single endeavor I have ever attempted – harder than college, marriage, child-raising, home ownership, high-paying jobs, managing people, talking with news reporters with my job on the line. Way harder.

Help improve the odds for your alcoholic or addict with much love and compassion from the start. Improving the odds for sobriety is important. Ultimately, addicts will be under the care of a counselor. I've never had a bad one. I had a few overwhelmed or under-trained counselors, but never one who didn't at least try. Counselors who don't care don't last in the business. Being a counselor is not easy.

I had superb counselors for each separate stay at AIA, beginning with the lead counselor, and ending with big Rick who woke me that first morning. To this day I quote from counselor No. 2, Matt, from something he repeated often straight from the big book of Alcoholics Anonymous: "Sometimes quickly, sometimes slowly, it will always materialize if we work for it." Me and several colleagues repeated this phrase to each other for years afterward. Some counselors like that take a Zen approach. Each has his or her own style. Regardless of their approach, almost all of them share with you this addiction problem. Even if they are clean or sober, most are still addicts, too. They're just much further along in recovery.

Rehab stays can be like college semesters. There's a set period of time, counselors, a curriculum, a significant amount of classroom sitting, a bit of recreation, and a lot of idle chat time. In the end, a sheet of paper, a pat on the fanny, and a "Good luck!"

Just kidding. At the end of rehab, you'll get, "Go straight to a meeting!" Phone numbers will be exchanged, promises made to keep in touch and help one another. A few might actually keep promises. That's actually a huge part of a successful treatment program: creating and nurturing a caring *support group*, and participating in what is called *after care*. Let's just say that for a decade, I skipped after care almost entirely. I did not do a formal after-care program like an IOP, and the results were unsurprising. When I tried my first IOP in 2021, I stayed sober almost two years. Note that. Some rehabs will attempt to keep in contact after you leave, but in my experience it doesn't last long.

A need for more assistance post-rehab, through that after-care period and into a sober living house or other outpatient program, is evident. More and more, it seems, rehab programs are opening their own sober living houses to continue care for the patients they just dedicated a considerable amount of energy trying to establish a foundation from which to work from.

That's really all rehabs do: help establish a foundation. I have never heard a rehab *promise a cure*, or anything like it. They're always clear there is no cure, and they cannot guarantee success, but they have a program or information to help you get started. The fact that recovery is a life-long mission is oft repeated.

* * *

From my first rehab, while only there 26 days, I wanted to offer a snapshot of some memories to provide a glimpse of what new rehabbers might expect. First, there were characters. There was a redneck drinker from Ohio who liked to poke fun at my single-strap backpack, calling it a purse. Due to this, years later, I laughed harder than I should have at the satchel scene in "The Hangover" movie. Later, I got revenge by diving up the middle as a shortstop in softball to rob him of a hit. Touche, redneck dude.

Earlier I mentioned the truck driver from Washington state living with me in the cabin. Another gentleman there, in fact my roommate, was an old guy from Houston who was extremely worried about losing his pension due to a drunken driving arrest. It didn't seem real that he could lose his whole public employment retirement just for a DUI. What was most memorable was he kept slipping on snow, falling so much he was issued old soccer cleats we found. It made for a heck of a visual, old jeans way above the ankles over black dusty plastic cleats. He also had some weird cabin habits, like peeing with the bathroom door open, or walking from the shower upstairs to our room with his ass hanging out the back, visible from us dudes sitting in the living room watching television. My friend Josh in particular would yell out at him to cover up.

An old van driver who later took Josh and I on a hairy snowstorm ride told the funniest story about his ex-wife, a lengthy dialog that ended with her floating around him in a room like a witch and him dodging her. Something like that. We always urged him to tell the story, and sometimes he'd do it in an AA meeting which made it even funnier. I loved that old guy, I think his name was John. I remember seeing him in his room (when he pinch-hit as overnight house manager) on his knees, hands clasped with head resting on the side of his bed, praying. He was deep into AA and very grateful to be sober.

There was this kid from Ohio who bragged a lot about bagging girls, whom Josh would somehow always manage to make sound stupid. A buff and well-tattooed dude was house manager for our connected cabins. Kind of a Dog the Bounty Hunter-looking character, but with shorter and more curly hair. He lived way down the mountain the other way, in Hesperia, with a baby at home to care for. There was Mark of Pennsylvania, who would meet up with me later, along with Josh, that year during my third visit.

A shocking discovery was seeing an old high school buddy sitting across from me one day in the Center's main room. We'd been sitting there a while, awaiting visitors, yet because I did not wear glasses my eyesight was blurry and I failed to make the connection. Eventually this dude's body mannerisms and curly hair tipped me off. "Glenn?" I asked. He looked at me weirdly. "Jajko?" (he probably most likely asked, "Polock?" A long-running joke). What a surprise. A young blond I met days prior by returning her lost jacket happened to be his daughter. What a look of confusion she gave when stepping into the room and seeing us talking about old times. She had no idea Glenn's brother, her uncle, is a very close friend of mine and has been for almost half a century. Glenn, too. We all surrendered a lot of brain cells together. I saw her again about seven years later, in a downtown Long Beach 7-11 store, where she worked as a side contractor for a tobacco marketer. I remember she intended to leave AIA with a dude from Long Beach, a guy we thought was bad news, and a place maybe not so desirable for recovery. She looked clean when I saw her at 7-11. She gave me Glenn's number. I never called, but see her smiling face on social media as she moved to Tennessee to be with her mother, who I also knew from school. It appears everything worked out.

Perhaps the biggest memory of a personality was Molly, an early-20s future mom from Ohio, up on the mountain to clean up for her mother. Just before she left program, we exchanged numbers while at an NA conference down the hill, and I remember how she phrased it when I said we should keep in touch and maybe see each other "on the outside." "*To go to a meeting*," she carefully clarified. I remember being at least a little disappointed, haha.

We never did use those phone numbers, but happened to connect on Facebook some time later. Still, we hardly conversed, until one day in mid-2024 I saw her post of a close-up shot of an NA chip, a logo I recognized. It had a lot of Roman numerals on it so I knew it was a biggie. Turned out to be Molly's 12th anniversary of being clean. She had remained clean the entire time since her last AIA stay. She would match me with three AIA stays that year, but she made sure those were her last rehabs. It was a miraculous story, and I messaged her to tell her so. By that time I had completed 12 rehabs, so I asked how she did it. Her direct words:

"It's been a helluva ride for sure. And hey, from the first time I went in 2012 in February to May, I ended up going back two other times. I thought I could do all the stuff I wasn't, because those were not my drugs of choice, but then I ended up coming back because Rick called and did a check-in. Honestly I don't know how I stayed, I just knew I couldn't get clean again if I went back out. I knew in my heart I'd never come back. So I've stayed away from everything for a long time. Everyone in my life today has never seen who I was. And I made a promise to my mom, she was my reason when I first got clean, and now I am a mom, and I don't ever want them to see me like that.

"AIA was life-changing. That part of my life was years I would never want to change. To be able to experience that, where we did in California in the mountains at the lake, all of it. So grateful for the people we've met along the way, and thankful for the ones who continue to stay around."

Molly ended or convo stating, "I haven't made it back to California yet but I plan to. My goal is to get up to Blue Jay [one of several small Lake Arrowhead communities] and spread my mom's ashes at the Rim of the World! I'll make it back one day." (She took a 13-year chip while I finished this book).

* * *

Besides the people, I saw some new and exciting stuff particularly the views and all the nature, and was able to make calls to begin the career clean-up. Once in the back of a white van returning from some night meeting, for whatever reason they comingled males and females. I was in the very back corner, two young (e.g. in their 20s) girls were in the seat before me, and Josh and another dude were in the next row up. For some reason someone dared the girls to smooch. So they did, kissing, open-mouthed and everything, right there between Josh and I. Josh doesn't recall, but I still chuckle thinking about it. (I asked Molly and she denied it was her, and I believe her; one of those gals ended up in Dana Point along the Orange County coast). I'm pretty sure before the smooch we were discussing favorite sex positions. I don't remember what I said, but I distinctly remember what Josh said: wheelbarrow! Good Lord, we all laughed hard. I don't know how the driver ignored us.

There was a big gym to visit weekly. This rehab had some killer deal with a fairly sizable gym in town, where we roamed free for a solid hour once a week, mostly by ourselves since it was during not-busy late morning time. The building was old but big with plenty of gear, and even had a racquetball court, where addicts could beat the shit out of each other with that small hard rubber ball. I would watch matches from a raised observation deck mainly to wait and see who would lose an eye. It was like watching car racing; I only watch for the crashes. I remember working out diligently on the machines and with dead weights. That started a trend where I exercised fairly hard at every rehab. Above It All was big on recreation and exercise, including some of the most memorable hikes ever experienced.

Career-wise, I had to call the director of the Free Clinic of Simi Valley, for which I served the board of directors, and also held a paying contract to fund-raise in an effort to get a new facility. I had to confess my location and reason for my absence. He was sympathetic, and said when I returned I had to tell the entire board at the next meeting I could attend. That ended up being one of the hardest things I've ever done. However, it went well, because after the raw emotion in the room during my brief speech, two board members spoke up and announced their two decades each of sobriety. You don't have to be alone in recovery.

Somehow I kept my main client, the national homebuilder, for the whole month simply by … doing nothing. I just lucked out with a quiet month; that project was in limbo awaiting big city hearings. They kept me on board because my mobile phone was the local 805 area code number for residents or the media to call for project-related information, and it just so happened that no one called. My wife kept my mobile phone and relayed messages. She visited once, and it was a long boring drive. I can't remember if she brought my phone that first time. She definitely did the second visit, because I was caught with it, really pissing off Dog the Bounty Hunter.

I remember being a pissant in some group sessions. Mostly silent and observant, I sometimes became instantly argumentative, or challenged group facilitators. When counselors hosted, I behaved; but had this tendency to give others a hard time. Maybe it was a carryover from my school days and substitute teachers. While really just a newbie to AA, I sure played the Big Shot know-it-all.

It's worth noting how I was not a typical first-time rehabber. By the time I entered AIA, I'd been with an addiction-specialist doctor for almost three years, and had attended a *lot* of AA meetings. I entered with an advantage over total newcomers. Josh and I came in with knowledge of AA, and it showed in meetings. We kind of showed off.

Finally one day I was stoned out. Program completers got nicely polished palm-sized stones with a single recovery-related word stamped on it. I'm pretty sure my counselor chose for that first ceremony a stone with "Peace" on it. Later I got one with "Hope." Can't remember the third but assume it's still stored with the remnants of my stuff with my mainland buddy Todd. I have a shoebox filled with those stones, along with a chain full of AA chips, everything from a newcomer welcome chip up to a nine-month chip. I don't remember getting a chip for the sole one-year ceremony I did, though it too could be at Todd's. When I almost reached two years sober I was not engaged with AA and got nothing, except periodic "Atta boy!" comments on IOP Zoom calls when I reached a milestone like 200 days, etc.

I look back on that first rehab and can honestly say it would have worked – *if I pursued, and adhered to, an after-care program.* Like many others, I left rehab to return directly to a home and job situation that had flared the problem in the first place. This despite constant reminders during program of the importance of attending a meeting immediately after discharge, getting a sponsor, doing the steps, doing the work needed to be healthy. It was a difficult lesson to learn. Hopefully, new rehabbers get it early. The period immediately after exiting rehab is crucial.

* * *

After meeting the nurse, some support staff, and your counselor, plus maybe a tour of facilities, the rehabber learns he or she will be living with a lot of strangers, few of them perfect church-goers. Rehabs are filled with friendly souls, many who are eager to help. It's not jail. Troublemakers are not tolerated; intimidation or threats result in ejection. Paid staff members are always near, most trained, many well-built physically.

You make a lot of friends in rehabs, because you share similarities, primarily a significant health issue that tends to cause the same problems in people. You might not meet them after treatment, or hang out much, but you *will* meet people with similar interests. For instance, I love punk rock, and befriended the former drummer for a fairly popular band from San Diego County, during my last AIA stay. His nephew, too, who is mentioned later in this book. I met a lot of baseball fanatics. You meet people from your hometown, from former places of residence, from your college.

Remember, you *all* begin with something big in common: addiction to mind-altering substances. A new rehabber doesn't have to say anything, yet he or she quickly will meet people with darn near the same situation. Losing kids to the government, or being on parole or probation, or difficulty avoiding cheap vodka – these circumstances connect strangers. This fact helps get past initial feelings of loneliness or pity. It's a big part of 12-step programs, to let you know you are not alone. Remember those first words from Rick on the detox couch. *You're in the right place.*

Gaining these friends and acquaintances is important. It's called your *support group*, and at AIA I noticed immediately a smart and witty former college football quarterback named Josh. Not only did I recognize his leadership among the boys during my first group sessions, I also got assigned to live in his cabin, the little four-bedder for older (more trustworthy, haha) clients.

In rehabs, they either take you to a lot of 12-step meetings, or they bring the meetings into your facility. My first rehab scheduled so many, one night a week they had us *run a meeting for ourselves*. No staffer or outside host. We chose a leader from among our group for each night. The leader would use AA's big book and manage the meeting like any other. Josh was selected for the first I attended at AIA. By this time I was well-versed with AA meetings; I'd attended meetings for several years before the rehab tours began. Eventually I, too, would be allowed to host and lead that meeting.

Most meetings were off-site, however. Lake Arrowhead has a small shopping center with a large drug store chain franchise, and two decently sized houses off to one side. The one on the right closet to the drug store is for hosting Alcoholics Anonymous meetings; next to it was for Narcotics Anonymous sessions. Every night. Probably some in daytime, too. In the classic white vans typical of treatment centers all over, the Center dropped us there often. It was a ritual, and honestly we didn't mind much, because it got us out and about, and also provided opportunity to see and be near the opposite sex. We might be troubled, but we weren't dead. In fact, sometimes I'd mix it up and attend a Narcotics Anonymous meeting, just for a change of scenery. To break the monotony, you might say. Inside, the NA meeting room seemed brighter. Plus, those meetings always seemed to attract a *lot more* females.

Early on, a couple of young 20-somethings were dickheads. One couldn't stop talking about all the girls he'd been with; the other just thought it was funny to drop rancid flatulence everywhere. We typically knew the latter was nearby because we smelled him. One night in the AA meeting house in Blue Jay (the name of the little subcommunity of Arrowhead), I sat directly behind Farter. Josh sat beside him, and a burly Indian-American was leading the meeting and he was quite serious. I noticed something off with Stinky; and saw Josh leaning over to whisper things in his ear and make motions indicating to *keep cool*. We alcoholics know when someone nearby is wasted, and when someone else is trying to help hide it. The sober guy kind of stiffens, and looks like he's acting. Josh was now playing that part. I saw Farter lean down to unzip his backpack on the ground between them, and point to something to show Josh, who quickly squished the bag shut. Josh told us later that Stinky showed off a big bottle of whiskey he'd nabbed from a team visit to the drug store earlier. (I learned to hate shit like that, because inevitably it would mean fewer store stops; always one dickhead to ruin it for the group).

In the meeting, the lanky kid overdid it. The group leader, the stocky guy with long black hair and plenty of tattoos, yelled for the boy to take his conversation outside, and stop disrupting the meeting. Then Fartmaster made a fateful choice. He stood up and yelled, "We were *talking program!*" At which the group leader yelled back and pointed to the door indicating to step outside, and briskly walked to his right and out the door. He was fiercely angry, and about 30 of us sat there eyes wide not knowing what to do. The kid froze, mumbled something, and sat down. Josh sat still as a statue. The leader came back, took a deep breath, returned to the dais, and apologized for his response. Then the meeting progressed without further incident.

That night upon returning to the cabins, we all had to pee in cups – known as urine analyses, or UAs. Everyone, a time-consuming process. Farter was not in our cabin so I didn't witness that scene. I could only imagine the ugliness. That shopping center meeting house is a very public place, pretty much known to anyone on the mountain attempting recovery. Long-timers there tolerate no nonsense; many of them don't even like the presence of rehabbers, but there's little they can do to stop it. After Fartmaster's explosion, without a doubt someone would call the program to report everything. A lot of long-timers there were so not fond of younguns with days of sobriety clogging *their* meetings, that an old leader would refuse to call on us to share, favoring only local friends. Anyway, the pee cups when we returned to the cabins proved we were very quickly snitched. Rehabs don't play around with public disturbances.

That program was located atop the large San Bernardino Mountains. It's high enough in elevation to host ski resorts in winter. In late spring, it's very cold at night. The program ejected Farter on the spot, returned his belongings, and kicked him out. Into the dark woods, at night, not far from a place named Big Bear for a reason. Farter got his cell phone back but being from Texas had no one locally to call. There was no Uber or Lyft in 2012, and I doubt a taxi at that time could have gotten him to Ontario Airport way down the mountain about 50 miles away. If he had the money for it.

Even though it was March, it still snowed often enough. I don't know what Stinky did that night or how he got home. I just remember the punishment seemed harsh. Lesson No. 3: put in street terms, *rehabs don't play*. In more modern terms, it might be *fuck around and find out*. Good ol' FAFO. Later I saw rehabs issue warnings or stern punishments for getting caught drinking or drugging, but they still let the culprit stay, albeit under special probationary terms. But not often. That might have been for dirty UAs. Being caught intoxicated on property, and especially with drugs, paraphernalia, or booze bottles, and your program ended. Many empty whiskey bottles were discovered over a back yard fence where Farter had been staying. It was enough for ejection.

Remember that my last stay at TTC – the same stint where I last saw my friend Ana – ended with me waking up in an emergency room. I returned from a pass blackout drunk and was immediately ejected. I also once chose to walk out of the Salvation Army after doing five months of the six-month program, after failing a pee test due to a single shot of tequila I found while working in the warehouse. For that one, I rejected an offer to surrender my 150 days of work, to begin anew at Day One. Even Rehab All-Stars make errors.

***

The rehabs I attended share commonalities. Most have the initial detox stay, a few days of maddening quietness interrupted too often by nurses to check vital signs, provide meds, or just ensure you're breathing. You spend a lot of time sleeping, broken up by many cigarette smoking breaks, and three meals. In my experiences, only the Salvation Army had no detox. It just had a rule requiring a potential captive to be at least five days clean and sober to get in. For which they had to take your word, a reason for my seizure at the beginning of my second stay. They do, however, use breathalyzer tests right at the front desk, and one time I crawled in for intake and blew a 0.06% blood-alcohol content the morning after a night of drinking. They sent me to sleep on the beach for hours before returning to try again. I got in, but ended up staying only a week. It would have been Sally stay No. 3. A single comment by the intake coordinator about a soon-opening winter shelter planted a seed that grew into a plan for a morning escape. I don't count that week as a rehab stay for this book.

Rehabs have rules and schedules. They all forbid the over-intermingling of the sexes (or even the same sex, if it's obvious). No violence, or even *threats or intimidation*, are tolerated. And of course no alcohol or drugs – in your system, on your person, in your living quarters, or anywhere on the property. As stated, having alcohol or a drug on property will get you kicked out. There are many other rules, both written and unwritten. So many that sometimes even staff members are unsure or unclear about them.

Some rehabs ban chewing tobacco (much to my chagrin in later rehabs); shaved heads; hats and/or hoodie sweatshirts; clothing glorifying alcohol or using; swearing; and other interactions. Some rules are anti-gang, or designed to keep faces clear for video cameras. Each facility required chores, usually daily, plus a monthly deep cleaning which for whatever reason they *all* call "double scrub." This is a period when everyone (supposedly) spends and hour or two at once cleaning spots oft ignored like inside or under refrigerators. This practice seems to get applied at sober living houses, too. Eventually I started asking myself, and anyone who would listen, if there are studies proving that chores make you any more sober or drug-free. My joke is that they all must read the same *Rehab Today* magazine, or something like it, and follow the same suggestions. A FOMO (fear of missing out) thing, or maybe they play Follow the Leader. Either that, or a memo goes out to all new rehabs and sober living houses dictating double scrubs. The uniformity is amusing.

These are all just *house* rules, or guidelines for living there. Actual rehabilitation *programs* vary in rules and structure, but they always involve a personal counselor, and a lot of time sitting among groups of peers. Sometimes groups get lectured at; other times, group members are asked to participate more. It depends on who facilitates (hosts) the group. Some are very good at it; some could care less; while for others it is something to endure. To each, his or her own. Group facilitators have great freedom in how they present information. There also are 12-step meetings, hosted by members of Alcoholics Anonymous, Narcotics Anonymous, and in one case at TTC, Cocaine Anonymous. They follow the 12 steps and rehabbers mostly get subjected to this at nights after a long day sitting in groups.

Program at the Salvation Army meant working 40 to 48 hours a week for pennies (literally $3 to $12 in cash weekly, plus coupons to use in a small canteen for food or snacks), in exchange for a bed, three daily meals, clothing, and other services like chapel. On top of all of this we were forced to attend at least four or five 12-step meetings a week. All told, it was a lot. However if you behaved, the Sally let you "check out" after work, like after 3 p.m., and stay out either four hours, or maybe even until 10 p.m. depending on the mood or administrators or desk volunteers. This privilege does not exist at other rehabs. Some rehabs have passes you can request to get out in the community, if you've been there a while and behaved. All allow passes for appointments like medical or legal. Most offer to connect you with resources like mental health services, and some like the Sally or Redgate in Long Beach encourage this. If you think you need special attention, just ask.

While the Sally program is all about the physical working aspect (they call it *work therapy*), other rehabs mostly have a schedule of daily groups, one or two hours focused on a single topic hosted by a counselor, program assistant (PA), or other staffer. Topics could include cognitive behavioral therapy, whatever that means. I've endured hours of CBT classes, and still can't explain it well. However, a psychiatrist once said that a tactic I applied to diffuse a tempting situation sounded like a CBT method. So maybe I got it by assmosis. It should be noted that you cannot out-smart addiction. In fact, being too smart, or overly inquisitive, can be a disadvantage. You can over-think or over-analyze, like my commentary on double scrub. I had a hard time not asking questions about why things were.

Other group topics might include life skills, orientation, family matters, etc. Some are physical education time like walking to a park, or playing volleyball. Some days get packed with hours of group sessions. Those are tiresome, though luckily mostly they allow plenty of breaks in between the sitting. It's noteworthy that rehabs can be paid for these group sessions, per signature. So rehabbers almost always hear right away from a group presenter, "Who has the sign-in sheet?" They've been trained to ensure getting those valuable signatures immediately, because gathering them later one at a time sucks. We tend to giggle when we see a group host walking around with a sign-in sheet looking for people.

Group topics can vary widely, and many are like what you see in the movie "28 Days" with Sandra Bullock. It could be "feelings," "personal journey," smoking cessation, co-occurring disorders, etc. Sometimes they get creative with topics; sometimes the facilitator's talks don't relate to the scheduled subject. Good rehabbers figure out which group presenters are fun, educational, to be tolerated, or dreadful. Since everyone goes by a weekly schedule, savvy rehabbers know to arrange appointments during times when sucky topics or facilitators are scheduled. Can't stand 120 minutes of culture weekly? Tell your counselor *that's the best time* for your weekly meeting. Beg if necessary. Savvy All-Star maneuver.

Rehabbers typically get some type of bookwork, or journal, that you're expected to complete to discharge. Some rehabs are more serious about this than others. Program work is usually easy, though young rehabbers can be great procrastinators, or even try to get others to do it for them. (It seems schools don't teach enough writing today). When writing is ordered, it's usually a *lot* of it, and you might find yourself carrying around a three-ring binder too much. Be prepared to write a lot with a pen. At TTC they would even call out "Pen check!" at the start of groups because having a writing instrument with you at all times was *required*. That was weird. You could get in trouble for not having a pen with you. It's all old-school homework, written out, since there's no mobile phones or word-processing computers.

It's part of what is known as The Program. In reality, it's *Your* Program, under the supervision and direction of *your* counselor. The groups supplement a syllabus, with the counselor meeting with you weekly to nudge along and monitor progress. Some counselors are good at helping meet life needs, like making calls the first few days when outside calls are disallowed; or providing coffee or goodies. Some are good at shooting the shit with you. I call this clock-eating and let them talk away. Some clients lean heavily on their counselor for all sorts of comfort. I was not among them, though I did get fairly close with some counselors. Some were just outright cool. Be assertive if necessary, and always remember it's *your* program, not theirs. Too often, we have to remind personnel who's boss. Clients pay the bills. No clients, no rehab, no counselor or staff paychecks.

That's essentially what to expect. Other than that, you will eat a lot, and usually above-average or even excellent food; and exercise. Outdoor activity was a huge part of the AIA program. Full-squad softball games (once with big Rick pitching), long and usually scenic hikes, free time at a local gym, or other white van excursions.

During my first AIA stay, we had a surprise late-winter or early spring storm that dumped many feet of snow everywhere. Our little old man's cabin was connected to the world by a little trail, to the bigger house with the house manager and white vans. For a day or more, the trail was buried under snow, and we couldn't locate it. It was long enough that we couldn't see the big cabin through the trees. One day, the Washington state truck driver went out and shoveled the whole darn thing. A great guy in his very first treatment program like myself, I learned not long after that he walked into the woods near his home and shot himself. It was my first experience with the death of a rehab colleague. More would follow, each time creating a solemn feeling that this shit was all very real.

This happened after every rehab. *Rehabbers who stray from recovery instructions can die.* Or go to prison. It should be eye-opening, but it hardly slowed me down. Years later at a sober living house on Maui, a 70-year-old on probation with multiple DUIs could recite AA slogans and steps by memory, but still decided drinking again seemed like a good idea. He was only "out" a day or so before the cops nabbed him. He got *five years in prison* for that. Ouch.

Still, while in rehabs, not everyone is always overly serious. One night during AIA No. 1, a program driver, who spent the night at the big cabin with the house manager enjoying time off, asked if anyone wanted to ride into town during a hellacious snowfall. Josh and I volunteered. It was the most nerve-racking short drive ever. First off, before we even got into the van, I slipped on snow at the van door and fell on my ass. Josh laughed *hard*. As we kept giggling in the van, the vehicle slid and swayed until we reached what the driver thought was a shortcut, downhill along a narrow street with cars parked along the side. Our target destination was Blue Jay and the drug store, but the residential street shortcut was on a steep slope, and though the driver inched down, it was clear we couldn't continue. The road was so icy, the driver returned us in reverse all the way back, taking advantage of tire tracks just crushed in the snow. Very slowly going backward, we somehow made it back to the cabin.

Not all rehab staff members do things like that. Some sneak stops at a store on a ride home, a nice treat. Sometimes they get caught. Some don't break rules because they'd already been caught and warned. Some staffers were just grouchy dickheads. Not many, but everyone knows who they are. For instance, during AIA stay No. 3, around October 2012, we started noticing penises, complete with huge balls and pubic hair, drawn onto van windows with a wet finger in the ever-present mountain dust. This seemed to go on for days, maybe even past a full week, and eventually the culprit used ink pens to leave penises on the underside of sun visors above the windshield, or once on the back of the headrest of a rear seat in an SUV used mostly to transport women.

Well one driver, let's call him Larry, noticed his rides seemed to get a lot of penises, and he complained to higher-ups. Now that I think about it, he might have been the *only* driver targeted with penises. Anyway, the permanent pen action on the SUV seat happened while he was driving, he reported it, and we were lectured that the culprit if caught would be charged the cost of cleanup. The head counselor was very perturbed, and in a nice way tried to get some of us to snitch. It's weird, but even new rehabbers know not to snitch. It's like it's become inbred in males over time. In reality, we did not know the culprit's identity.

A short time later, at night while we all hung out in the big cabin's living room, the discussion swerved to the penises. Who was this mysterious penis-maker? Who was this bold soul who left penises with balls and pubic hairs in his wake? Usually on or inside Larry's vehicles? An excellent rehab conversation. Finally after some time, we heard from a corner a calm, "I did it." Our punk rock drummer who says he's from Andromeda shrugged and said, "Larry's a dick." We all laughed, mainly because we agreed, and that was that. In all honesty, it could have been any one of us in the room.

The next day, Larry backed a white van between two other vans to park, and walked into the Center, where we had groups or lunch upstairs. Just prior, clients congregated and smoked or chewed tobacco outside an exterior staircase. I noticed Larry walking from his van around the side of the building to an office entry. I am rarely late for meetings, but I watched as guys and gals one at a time went up those stairs. Once alone, I meandered (probably even tip-toed like some cartoon character) over to the vehicle lineup and walked behind Larry's dusty van, licked a finger, and drew a huge penis complete with huge balls and pubic hair on one of the rear windows. Then I went up to the meeting.

And sometimes I wonder why my rehabs don't stick. Looking back, I did goof off too much, beginning at the first rehab. It's hard not to, in my opinion. Rehab life can be monotonous. An AA book says somewhere to not take ourselves so damn seriously. Rule 62. Look it up. I can find no other AA "rules." That's how much AA believed in Rule 62. They made no other rules to cloud the issue.

* * *

I was informed I had 28 days each time I walked into AIA. The first time, I took a completion letter at 26 days, claiming it was the only day I could get a ride home, which may have been true. Just before leaving that first time, they provided a form for feedback. I filled it up, being the ego-crazed writer that I was, telling them *how precisely to run a rehab*. No appreciation, which I regret. At each rehab stop, I learned a little more to be grateful, and try to limit whining about the program. It's vital to remain in a state of gratefulness as much as possible. After all, I was lucky to be alive. Still am. New rehabbers should remind themselves often how lucky they are for their rehab bed.

After those 26 days, I stayed sober about another 50 days, for about 75 total. Arriving home, I didn't immediately hit a 12-step meeting as recommended, but I did consistently attend an early-morning meeting not far away in Simi Valley. I didn't go every day, but often, getting done by 7:30 a.m. to get back home to drive my son to high school.

Then, in my infinite wisdom, I decided to take that son, and his classmate friend, both age 13, to a three-day punk rock music festival in Las Vegas over Memorial Day weekend. What possibly could go wrong? It proved I did not listen properly in all those hours of rehab therapy. That relapse was a slow-roller, like a little pebble on an extended slope that started rolling downhill and grew larger and larger until it was a huge unstoppable ball. By September, my wife drove me back up the mountain for another stay at AIA. Oh how I wish the second rehab had stuck, but after only 27 days I claimed work demands and got out. *Just eight days later*, at the beginning of October, my father drove me back up the mountain for a third AIA attempt. Memories of the last two AIA programs sometimes blur, so apologies if some details seem off. For No. 2, I had a counselor named Matt. Their rule was to assign a new counselor for returnees. Matt was pretty darn good, very mellow and spiritual, always giving sound advice, sometimes right from AA literature. When I got back for stay No. 3, my counselor was big Rick mentioned earlier.

* * *

AIA No. 2 began around the first week of September 2012. Pretty much immediately I started thinking about exiting. Once again, I left early, but just by a day, for "work." Which by then amounted to just the controversial housing development in my hometown. I might have had a content article writing assignment or two, but … The wife now had a job, but we weren't covering the mortgage. We had pre-teen daughters in expensive competitive cheer, and a son into the bass guitar, a modest drum kit, and video games. While expenses increased, here was dad, in rehab, limiting income. The wife again drove me to the top of the mountain and left me at AIA.

After I survived my second experience with detox, I met young Zach, who I saw walk into the smaller detox center, which was adjacent to the first place they assigned me to, not really a separate cabin but more of a regular house right on the Rim of the World highway. The house was split in half, detox on one side surrounded by a huge wood deck overlooking the woods, and our living quarters opposite. I didn't like the house manager there, who I remember from stay No. 1 (an aging gang-banger), and within a week I weaseled my way into the same small cabin as before. Looking back, it hints at an ego gone wild, to even make such a request. The Big Shot bullshit mentioned in the AA book, another hint that I was not grasping concepts needed to recover. That is, humility is huge.

Before leaving that new home, I could walk around the big deck around detox to sit and smoke, and watch new arrivals crawling outside for fresh air or quiet time. The only one I remember is Zach. He sat alone at a big round table, posture slumped, eyes almost shut, sick as shit. Coming down off heroin or opiates, Zach was hardly in the shape to talk. But we hit it off somehow; maybe I had smokes to offer, I don't remember. It wasn't until way later in that stay that we started talking punk rock. I'm confident that I brought along a Social Distortion tee that I wore often – and he mentioned his uncle played drums for a known band from San Diego County. That did not register until I returned for AIA No. 3, because by that stay his uncle was there with Zach and I.

***

I spoke with Zach over the phone in August 2025, and here's snippets of his memories with AIA, and also thoughts about relapses and maintaining sobriety. Zach said he'd been to 16 inpatient treatments, *half* of those at AIA. Eight visits to one rehab! A true Rehab All-Star. He shared many of my own experiences, including multiple sober living houses, and discovering just how awful other facilities can be after AIA.

At one point he was over four years clean, had worked up to a restaurant manager's position, and lived in a place overlooking Newport Harbor. He was cruising and loving life. Then old habits returned and would not go away. "I pretty much lost it. I went into a meltdown-induced psychosis," Zach said.

Ultimately his mother tricked him into seeking help by saying she believed he had a stroke, that he was slurring words and that part of his face drooped. Seeking medical attention, he was informed that his liver and kidneys were failing. He survived, and moved into a sober living house, where he stayed nine months. He had a close call at just eight days there when his beloved grandmother passed, but his mother and a sober living house manager helped convince him to stay, plus luckily he was involved with an outpatient program for support. "I wanted to run, but my mom begged me to stay," he said. "So I stayed, and it drained me."

We talked some about being rehab wizards, and playing the Big Shot. "I would say, 'I could be the counselor here, or the therapist.' And it's not a good thing to say, to even think," Zach said. "You should have shut the fuck up and absorbed everything, instead of goofing off, and treating it like a vacation."

On his experiences with AIA, Zach has fond memories, especially when compared against what followed. "At AIA were some of the best managers I ever had. We had the most solid, awesome group you can have in rehab. There's nothing that has been close to matching that. The crew was so solid."

By August 2025 he had been in his own apartment for seven months, skipping the sober living houses. He knows the inpatient rehab stuff well, and says it's just a matter of putting in the work and effort. Nonetheless, he fears relapse and where it might land him. "It gets worse every time. You just don't realize just how good you had it at AIA. They did everything for us, and we took it for granted. I've learned to be grateful for a lot of things, little things even."

Sound familiar?

* * *

Honestly, I have the fewest memories of AIA No. 2 than other rehab stays. Perhaps because Nos. 1 and 3 had so many big things happen – first detox, first rehab, and later softball with my own gear, hikes with Zach and his uncle and others, Josh returned, wife and family fled, etc. During AIA No. 2, I remember living with two really big guys in that small cabin. One was a former college football lineman from the San Francisco Bay area, and the other was from Bakersfield obsessed about fighting. There's a photo around somewhere of me outside the cabin wearing the Social D shirt sandwiched between those giants. Good guys, I hope they made it.

This was my first experience as a "return customer" at a facility, and I quickly went into "Been there, done that" mode. This was unfortunate, not only at that moment but also later at revisited facilities. I didn't pay enough attention to lessons, and failed to double down on effort. Instead of punishing myself for failing, I coasted. To put it in sports terms, I watched the clock. I believed I was ahead and winning, and that little could be done to change that. I either underestimated or misjudged the power of my addiction. It was a very costly mistake I'd make repeatedly, and I hope anyone reading this avoids. I lost a lot of income from all these visits, but more importantly, a lot of time, and respect. Time lost with my kids, and family members, and friends. I didn't know it, but I was starting a very slow and long period of withdrawal from the society I knew for three-plus decades. Sobriety aside, I'd already changed. I was now this aging former professional battling a life-threatening ailment. All the AA, therapy, and rehabs had changed how I perceived life and happenings around me. Much more change was to come.

Perhaps the biggest memory of AIA No. 2 was a physical reaction to a medication given to help with sleep. Early that year, I was prescribed Trazodone, and had been taking it many months and it seemed to help. While the side effects warning mentioned potential for prolonged erections, it said they would last *up to* four hours. Indeed, at home I had some mornings with surprise wood, but walked it away. However, early in this rehab stint, one morning walking wasn't enough. It was alarming when the call came to walk to the van for transport to the Center and groups. I put on a big baggy hoodie and stretched the bottom down to below the waistline, so I could pull it down to cover my crotch as I walked with my hands in the front pouch. I would be squished in with dudes in the van, and I hoped the boner would not get discovered. I prayed for it to go away.

It didn't. I somehow was able to walk from the van into the Center, and sat through the first group. Eventually I was bent forward a bit, half to hide it, but also because it started hurting. It raged so long at full-bore that it was painfully full of blood. I braved the group, and during a break before the next group, I trudged to the nearby office of my first counselor. "I have an erection that won't go away," I explained, shaking my head. "It's stuck." His initial reaction was amusement, as if he'd heard a *lot* in rehab over the years, but *never this*. But he quickly caught himself, properly identified the emergency, and called for an immediate ride to the little medical center atop the mountain. That made for a second embarrassing conversation, with the driver. (It was not Larry). "Why don't you just, you know, like, take care of it?" he said, with a hand gesture hinting at what I already knew he suggested. I replied, "I can't even touch it. It's too painful!"

Which led to embarrassing moment No. 3: the ER front desk. I explained what happened, and the desk lady quickly snickered aloud a little but caught herself to at least keep a straight face going forward. I felt like the "Biggus Dickus" scene in the Monty Python movie, trying to talk to people without them laughing. Luckily, the ER doctor arrived and acknowledged the seriousness of the situation, and I was very quickly escorted to a bed inside a curtained cubicle area. Unfortunately, there were no urologists nearby, no specialists, and due to the time crunch involved (I learned later if blood accumulates there too long cells could be damaged) he would have to try to resolve it. But, how? By applying … what? Tips from a med school course he remembered?

Tacking on to my experience was embarrassment No. 4. After I stripped and lay there naked with my boner pointing to my belly button, the doc brought in two interns to watch the procedure. Two *young women*. I'm not sure if he asked for my approval, but by this time my mind was like, "*How could this possibly get any worse?*" And, "*I just want this hard-on gone!*" So we forged ahead.

Basically, he poked a hole on either side of my penis, kind of near the centerpoint, and hand-squeezed the blood out. I don't remember any pain killers, and I most definitely was awake. I felt like Sir Gallahad the Pure in Monty Python's "Holy Grail" film, with people poking around my pecker as I laid there looking at the ceiling, eyes darting back and forth. Maybe my dick was numb by that point. It took maybe 10 minutes, then they left and let me lay there atop a pool of thick red-brown blood that had dripped down around my body and pooled underneath my butt. There was a *lot* of very dark blood. I repeat this often: *you learn a lot in rehabs*. I learned a heck of a lot about how erections form, held, and if necessary drained.

It was a great relief to get out of there and back to civilization and our groups. I was honest with the guys about it, laughingly explaining it in detail. From that point on, my nickname was Kickstand.

The ordeal stretched into the next morning for embarrassment No. 5. Overnight, my penis turned colors, apparently from bruising above and below the incision points, or the squeezing. The result was a flaccid phallus that looked like a two-toned ice pop as a child – brown on the ends, and a light yellow in the center. Like it bruised at the base and near the tip where doc GI Joe Kung Fu Grip squeezed and twisted. Early in group the next day, I was called in to see the program's contract nurse. For some reason someone decided a follow-up was necessary. (I bet it was a joke arranged by staff, maybe because I'd made fun of someone). She immediately asked me to pull down my shorts so she could inspect the, ahem, specimen. I think she actually used that word, specimen. I pulled down my shorts and underwear, and stood. She was sitting, so everything was there right in front of her face. So here, this middle-aged stranger carefully pinched the head between her thumb and index finger, to lift it up away from my body. She ducked her head low, and very close to it, for a truly close inspection. She squinted her eyes and seemed amused by the coloring, and looked closely at the tiny incision points. I don't know why it was necessary, but I didn't mind. It just added to the legend. (Side note: one night in 2014 I absentmindedly accepted from a girlfriend a "sleeping pill" without asking about it. I was desperate for good rest. The next morning, we went through the same drill at an ER in Simi Valley. This time they called in a urologist to do the penis puncturing and squeezing. My girlfriend giggled from behind a curtain the entire time.)

* * *

I did 27 days that second rehab stay – and remember being proud of myself for staying *longer* this time. One frickin' day. Once again I asked to leave early for "work," which still was just a single client and maybe a project or two. At the beginning, once again I was assigned to the small cabin for old guys. I remember Rick hosting a group there once, and that it was memorably funny. Zach mentioned repeatedly that his uncle is the drummer for a punk band. (Who I would meet my next AIA stay). I lived with the two huge guys. We played more softball, and I made a mental note to bring equipment "next time." In the middle, I was caught with my iPhone, which would be impactful for AIA No. 3. Eventually, I stoned out of AIA No. 2, and the wife came for me. I would be back within days.

* * *

With **AIA Stay No. 3**, October into November 2012, I was determined to "finish" the program, to complete the entire 28 days. Honestly I didn't have anything better to do. During stay No. 3, my wife packed up the house and took everything of value in it along with the kids and even cats to Missouri, and put the house up for sale. Getting out of the mortgage was like shrugging a boulder off my back, the relief so large. My brain was not yet working properly and I didn't truly ascertain what happened. My wife and kids were moving almost 1,700 miles away, to be closer to the wife's aging mother, and the house I owned would be sold. I would be homeless soon, and didn't understand the ramifications.

* * *

I can't adequately explain how embarrassing it is to return to the same rehab after being gone a short time. Guys who just watched you graduate are still there. This time my wife deferred the drive to Dad, and along the way came his "Treat it like an adventure!" speech. Finally up there, entering the little intake room in the basement of the big detox, a guy from stay No. 2 happened to walk in. "Hey Keith!" he almost yelled. Then, his eyes widened as he realized I was *back*, and that my presence was not a positive thing. "Ohhh," he stammered, nodded knowingly, and exited fast.

This visit was unlike the previous, mainly because the wife put the house up for sale and would move to Missouri, where she came from in 1988 (and immediately met me). Upon leaving AIA, I could start afresh, so I thought. Certainly, erasing the mortgage was a palpable relief.

During this stay, I developed solid friendships, with dudes like Zach and his uncle, plus a huffer from San Diego, and a guy we nicknamed Sandy from Arizona. Later, Josh and a returnee from Pennsylvania from my first stay returned, and both were assigned to my room.

This time I brought my softball gear, and we had serious games. Zach and his uncle had hilarious stories. The cool San Diego dude was the first person I met addicted to *huffing* – inhaling fumes from computer cleaner spray cans. His story of getting a DUI while driving blacked-out on a freeway on-ramp was impressive. I doubt I'll ever hear that one again. You hear a lot of *firsts* stories in rehab. Many are quite insane. Eventually nothing surprises you. Do rehab enough and eventually your stories become a first for some newbie. Not a status you want to attain.

Early on, maybe the first day, we had a van ride to Joshua Tree National Park. It was a nice trip, and we hiked a short distance up some big standstone rocks. We sat down and had a "process" group with counselors Rick and Ron. Rick, the big guy who woke me the very first morning at AIA, was assigned my program overseer this time.

Somehow the group discussion delved into AA and, particularly, the higher power concept, and I had a meltdown. After a few dudes shared, I just blurted out something like, "AA relies on voodoo!" To which the punk rock drummer shrugged his shoulders and calmly said, "I like voodoo." Counselor Ron and I exchanged words, and his input was heartfelt, but my mind was stuck. After the session we mingled about outside the van, and I sat alone on a curb. Rick approached and asked what was wrong, and going by memory I said I was sick of AA. He comforted me somehow, and I don't remember what he said, but it convinced me to at least try one more time. Again, for returnees, early on it's hard to get past thoughts of all the group sitting to come.

For this last AIA stay, I stayed 32 days, and actually worked with the program to arrange for more time in a sober living house down the mountain in Upland. There, I learned this two-story residential home holding like a dozen of us was not a sober living house, but in reality another residential rehab program. We rarely left the house, sitting in groups all day, and they had an in-house cook for meals so we even ate right there in the same living-dining room. We did at times get driven into town for abbreviated gym time, but nothing like AIA. My counselor was kind of weird, the main manager guy wasn't overly helpful, and I got annoyed at a staffer who started God-lecturing while we sat at the Thanksgiving table. I barked at him hard, that meal times were *our* time, and that we'd appreciate a break from all the lecturing. The guys loved me for that, and after the meal I called my parents and asked Dad to come get me. I'd been there 10 days, and it was a rehab and not sober living program. As I waited in the living room for the ride, the same lecturing staffer was finishing his shift, and he stopped briefly and just said, "I'll pray for you."

At the time I took it as a dis (for disrespect), but years later found myself saying the same thing to folks in recovery who I had friction with, or who somehow seemed troubled. We addicts can be short-tempered (surprise!). During those moments, anyone nearby gets stress from a blowup. Experienced people will know what to *not do*. That is, do not lecture, or scold, and otherwise overly try to calm. Just politely say something like that above, or "take it easy," or another AA cliche phrase, and move on. Blowups pass.

I arrived home to a house empty of family, of any life or love, really. I did however have my parents two houses away, which helped some. Still, I relapsed within days, and by mid-December was banished from my parents to live in my old house with no water or power. I have no idea what I ate during this period, only that a woman friend was delivering vodka now and then. I was basically waiting around to die.

My parents must have sensed something, because one day as I was half through with a fifth of vodka, Dad entered the house's front door and yelled for me. I heard him from my old room. "Keith, come eat," he ordered. After finishing off most of the vodka and carefully hiding the bottle, I did.

They fed me well and asked me to stay there. I asked that they monitor me as I detoxed. I reached a point where I knew what came after each heavy drinking bout. I knew I'd be ill. I did fairly well through the holidays, even attending meetings for SMART Recovery, kind of a modernized version of AA, minus the spiritual angle. I was trying new things, something I still do. Who knows what might work for each individual? The woman who'd been supplying vodka and hanging out at my house some nights relapsed and soon went to a 90-day treatment program in the Valley. Then I was truly on my own. I lasted sober until about Jan. 11, 2013, when a memorial was held at a nightclub for an old friend they found dead in a riverbed in Oxnard. A suspected overdose, possibly heroin, and maybe done purposely by bad people. His older brother, who I knew even better, already years before had shot himself in Georgia. I drank heavily at the nightclub memorial and got a ride home, and the next morning my parents noticed my truck missing. It was at the nightclub, and I couldn't explain why. I walked miles to the club to get my truck, Tapo to First Street, and returned to my house to complete a few weeks of sheer Hell, saved only by a client-friend and his pastor who trekked to Barstow to rescue me from a tiny motel room. Those details are not rehab-related and are for another time, maybe a follow-up book. Needless to say, the three rehabs of 2012 were for naught.

* * *

Josh returned in the middle of my third AIA stay. When he arrived in the small detox, my first counselor found me and offered to drive me there to see him and offer encouragement. Josh wasn't doing well, I was told. I walked in and he saw me, and I'm unsure whether he recognized me. He looked terrible, eyes glazed, and a real sad look on his face. Eventually we hugged, and I said I was there for him once they moved him over to a cabin.

He wasn't the same person from AIA No. 1. Earlier in the year he was quite funny, smart, at times spiritual, even prophetic. Now, you could sense deep sadness and regret. His wife, his high school sweetheart and mother of three young children, was not returning. Josh struggled fiercely with that for the final two weeks we were together in the big cabin. By this time I was in the bigger cabin, and they assigned him to room with me. Soon after, a colleague from AIA No. 1 joined us, a dude from Pennsylvania. I was assigned to that cabin to keep close to the house manager, since during the previous stay my iPhone was discovered and confiscated.

So, three return customers in the same room. Minor league rehab all-stars. I didn't realize it then, but those guys would "get it" and would avoid promotion to the major-league Rehab All-Star status of Zach and I. Certainly Josh didn't stay clean the entire time. He called me in spring 2016 asking to borrow some dough, which I provided. We spoke at length one evening as I prepared dinner in a central Long Beach sober living house, and he was too chatty to be clean. At the time I was over a year sober, starting with the 10 months at the Salvation Army and extended at a house with other Sally survivors. It sounded like he was struggling, but I said nothing. Josh asked for $65, which I knew was around the price of an eight ball, or eighth of an ounce, of meth. And he was living in an area far from his home in north Central Valley, down in a dry dusty area outside Los Angeles with a reputation for … meth.

No matter, I had the money, with a friend in need. It's just how I am, and I'm sure it was the same for those who sent me dough over the years. I worked out some kind of phone app transfer while waiting at the Willowbrook station of L.A.'s Metro Blue Line, mid-commute to a middle management job marketing for a national custom closet manufacturer in south-central L.A. Josh messaged me a thank you, and that was the last we discussed it.

Years later I would see him smiling big on Facebook, with a new girlfriend, who he eventually married and settled with in the San Gabriel Valley area. Those eyes I knew from the first AIA stay had returned, and I was stoked for him. I had a pretty solid feeling Josh would make it, despite the early struggles in Arrowhead and Beaumont. He was close with Christ, and I was confident he wouldn't stray far. Spirituality is helpful in recovery. It allows the afflicted to dedicate energy to something, which in turn helps get the addict out of his or her own head. Spirituality can provide hope when it seems little is coming.

I'm unsure whether Josh (or our Pennsylvania friend) had a third rehab stay. They definitely did not do even half the number of rehabs I tested. I can't call Josh a major league Rehab All-Star. However, those guys spent time in the minors.

Other memories of the last AIA visit include free bowling with pizza and sodas on Saturday nights; Sunday movies at a theater; and a field trip to Griffith Park above downtown Los Angeles, where our punk rock drummer did something I still recall with great amusement. He said he was from Andromeda, a planet far out in space, and we kind of believed him. He had a gigantic alien face tattoo covering his entire back, after all. At Griffith Park, we learned that, just maybe, it was more than just an obsession.

When we arrived and parked, painted on the concrete as you approached were arcs indicating the orbit of each Solar System planet, around the observatory as if it was our sun. We started walking to the observatory, but the drummer put his head down like a bloodhound and raced ahead as if in search of something very important. He disappeared into the building, and it took a few minutes before we caught up inside. Upon arrival, we saw this huge time-keeping pendulum in the center of the lobby, rocking rhythmically back and forth keeping time, a wondrous sight. Just as we were getting acquainted with the main room and doors to side rooms, we heard the drummer yell out, "There it is! There it is!"

We hustled to turn a corner, and saw him pointing excitedly at a big display that showed galaxies around ours. "Andromeda!" he yelled and pointed. Sure as shit, shown and listed right there, was Andromeda. It was a real place, after all.

At the end of my AIA stay, I felt different, as if I too was from another planet.

PART TWO

CHAPTER 3

TARZANA TREATMENT CENTER NO. 1 AUGUST TO NOVEMBER 2013

Welcome to the Jungle

I was unaware future rehabs would differ from Above It All. It shouldn't have been surprising. When I later thought about it, being atop a mountain in the cool clean woods living in well-supplied cabins was like a summer camp experience – not a more strict or punitive setting you might expect from a place focused on serious substance abuse matters. For me, the latter was coming.

There also were big changes developing in the treatment universe, something I didn't realize until years later. I just happened to experience my recovery journey during a period when the rehab industry would be altered considerably, due to regulatory changes and the market's response. Think about it: I've experienced rehabs both *before and after* the Affordable Care Act, commonly called Obamacare. This national health care edict became law in 2010, but full implementation lasted to 2014. By that year, I had completed four stays at two different rehabs. The ACA mandates that most health plans cover behavioral health services, including treatment for substance abuse disorder. It was momentous for rehabs.

My stints in AIA occurred in 2013 and 2018, first in late winter-early spring, then late summer into early November. Since my wife worked in government, I had good health insurance, so probably none of this mattered at the time of early ACA implementation. On the last day of July 2013, I entered Tarzana Treatment Center on the north side of the San Fernando Valley. It provided an opportunity to witness changes that seemed to start with the ACA. To the point: not many share my experiences, first in a private treatment program, then in publicly funded care.

Back in 2012, most rehabbers had to be wealthy or have good insurance to get treatment for abuse of alcohol or drugs. It's a reason over the years we mostly heard about rehabs when celebrities or the super-rich participated. They could afford it. I would venture to say most Americans could not. For instance, as late as 2012, AIA charged $30,000 a month, or $1K a day. My insurance pitched in $15,000, and AIA *chose* to cover the rest. It did not have to. In one of my stays, the daughter of a high school buddy attended. Her AIA rehab was privately funded by my friend's brother, whom I was even more close with as a friend. She was young and trying to kick heroin. Heck of an uncle, I'd say, to pony up thousands of dollars for just a month of treatment.

How many United States residents in 2012 could afford to skip 30 days of work, and pay $30,000 (or more), for treatment? Over the years thousands, if not millions, of Americans did not get inpatient treatment for abuse of alcohol or drugs. The ACA helped open the door for more people to get help. The challenge of finding open rehab beds quickly might remain; many have waiting lists that can stretch to many weeks. Sometimes it's just the pure luck of timing when you call, or walk in a door. Other times, it's who you know. That's how I got into Tarzana without waiting. Twice, in 2013 and 2018, exactly five years apart, with help from different friends. No need to get into the strings pulled, but let's just say I have a *lot* of friends, dating back to my school days. It helps that the rehab industry has grown so large, that if you know a lot of people, there's a decent chance you know someone who works for a rehab. Gone are the days where rehabs were mostly exclusive getaways along the coast.

Some people may still have that perception, but it's not what I got at Tarzana, known as TTC. What I remember at TTC, even early on, was the fact that pretty much the entire time I was there I complained about it. I sure learned a hard lesson about gratefulness. I discovered that AIA was

Camp Snoopy compared with alternatives. Lake Arrowhead was beautiful, the accommodations cozy, the experience an adventure, as my father had hoped. A solid environment and vibe to establish recovery.

At Tarzana, since the wife moved away and I had no insurance in 2013, I received what was called a "county" bed. That is, a bed funded by the county government and free for me, which could have been linked to the ACA, maybe not. It probably was just part of an agreement for the larger parent corporation to provide some charity services, in exchange for something they really wanted like a big contract to provide regular health clinics elsewhere. I ended up in a dorm of six bunks, with 12 beds total, mostly full all the time. I don't remember beds being empty for long. Not all TTC rooms were like that. They had some two-, three-, and maybe four-bed rooms, but those seemed reserved for paying customers, whether private pay or insurance.

Besides the smaller rooms, there were three male-only dorms. My first experience living in a room with 11 other people. There was another dorm on the other side of the building, where I stayed in 2018, with seven bunk beds. Beyond that, adjacent and accessible only by walking through the just-mentioned 14-bed dorm room, was *another* 14-bed dorm. Mind you, these rooms were not particularly large. Essentially it was barracks living, big time, 40 troubled males in all packed into not a lot of space.

I remember my thoughts when walking the crowded halls on the transfer from detox into residential. "Wow, this place is packed." Followed by, not long after, "This place *sucks!*" Luckily I was assigned to a bottom bunk in a corner of the room, a prime location. I was awarded a bottom bunk due to high blood pressure, seriously pissing off the bed's previous inhabitant who happened to have ram horns tattooed on the sides of his shaved head. He got moved to an upper bed near the door directly under a big fluorescent lighting fixture. It was akin to a jail bed, constantly staring up at a bright light, so let's just say he was pissed. Of course, I was blamed. Not a promising start. Eleven roommates, without our own bathroom. For that, we shared a restroom a good

200 feet or more down a hallway, publicly open for anyone in the entire facility to use. It had three shower stalls, two sinks with mirrors, and two toilet stalls.

I learned that's what you got for free, and I was thankful. I quickly realized the value of my wife's job and its insurance. Thinking back to my friend Ana from this book's first story, I remember she was in a two-bed room, but only for 14 days. I honestly think she could have requested an extension. Her husband was a police officer, with above-average insurance most likely. The program would have considered allowing more time, if insurance approved it. With rehabs, in my experience, finances (whether it meant spending, or potentially enhancing revenue, if you will) greatly influenced the decision-making process.

At TTC, the detox and group sessions were pretty much the same as at AIA. What was new for me was everything in the same, single facility. There wouldn't be van rides every day. Not often, but sometimes, we got rides to and back from nighttime AA meetings. The TTC campus was all concrete and asphalt, thickly carpeted hallways, and a single big tree out back for some shade. Indoors, it had a hospital vibe. Maybe even, to some extent, the feel of a hospice.

There were two sizable houses for detox centers at AIA, and you can imagine the setting. Multi-bed rooms, of course, but also living rooms with reading materials and television, plus great meals cooked on the spot. You lived large for a few days in detox at AIA, which is nice when your brain is foggy, body exhausted, and gait unsteady.

The two detox centers at TTC were more straight-up hospital settings. The first time there, I was in a decently sized detox with access to the outdoors, in fact a huge quad area with grass, table seating, a ping-pong table, and pay telephone. In 2013, I didn't know anything about the other detox center there. I learned in 2018. It was beds separated by curtains, and a small cage area for mingling and smoking. I'm fairly certain there was a ping-pong table. That's it. Every once in a while we might be allowed out onto the grassy quad, but not often, and only for brief periods. Mostly I remember all the nonstop smoking in the cage, and whining by an opiate withdrawal victim who pined for Suboxone. (In 2018 and 2019 I'd have similar detox experiences in Long Beach; both facilities had above-par nurses and medical care inside rather limited environments).

Tarzana was a big campus, much larger than that of Redgate in Long Beach later on, which is quite small and looked like a former nursing home or senior citizens care facility. Tarzana had that vibe too, but there was much more there. A swimming pool in the back, next to a small tent-like room that served as a gym, and a decent-sized asphalted back area with a ping-pong table and plenty of seating. Indoors, there were long hallways, two straight, connected by a curving one where they housed women or young mothers with children. We had to be quiet walking the middle hallway. That curved passageway encircled the rear end of a massive dining area, with a long kitchen stretched out because meals were buffet style. That was rather nice, where you slid a tray down a rail shelf and loaded up with whatever you wanted. You could eat a lot during TTC meals, that's for sure. Coffee included during mornings, but like Redgate, not after noon. Unlike Redgate, TTC's dining area was always open, so you could swing by for juice if you wished. They had huge flowing containers you could see inside, a rainbow of enticing flavors. Or, to have quiet time to read, study, or write. Experienced rehabbers know the value of finding places to hide away, for mental health breaks. It can be draining being around strangers all the time, and addicts at that. The chatter seemed constant.

Tarzana was crowded in 2013, and it was way worse in 2018. I'd estimate they nearly doubled the population by 2018. I suspect it was because it was a large corporation, with another substance abuse clinic in Long Beach, and also numerous regular health clinics funded by the county. It appeared the corporation chased government reimbursement dollars. Whether from the county or, most likely, the larger government entities, you know they logged every action or service provided to get to their accounting offices to bill government or insurance companies. The place in 2018 was day-and-night compared with the first stay; I'll get to that troubled second stay later. It was unbelievable to see, honestly. I guess understandable when excessive government funding is available ready for the taking, and you happen to have a big operation already established where you can squeeze in a lot of people, with the administrative infrastructure already in place to manage it all. Today, rehabs can get funding for pretty much anything they do. Some take it to the extreme. But I digress.

I can't say if that's good or bad. It means more people than ever can get professional help for addiction, or other mental ailments. In fact, today anyone can get into a treatment program. They will take the uninsured, which they might have done pre-ACA, but not in bulk. With the ACA, at least in some states like California and Hawaii, a rehab can get the client insured on the spot to take them in. I think some rehabs take pretty much anybody, and then work to get reimbursement somehow. Sometimes it works 100%, but as I learned with AIA, some could be willing to take half the compensation they typically demand.

Here is a broad look at the rehab industry; more on my TTC stays later. It's the only rehab I never completed. It's also the only rehab that never provided an exit date to target.

* * *

Until the 1940s, chronic alcoholics had little hope. It was worse for drug addicts, but then there weren't near as many, at least that we knew about. In the past, most drug users hid from society. Drugs were much more seriously frowned upon before the 1960s. Even for decades after, few would admit to being involved with heroin or opiates. With the epidemic created by the pharmaceutical industry this century, opioid abuse is much more known and, to an extent, accepted. American society still has not come to terms with the seriousness of the fentanyl crisis.

Back in the 1940s, all chronic alcoholics and addicts had was stays in hospitals, and maybe doctor-prescribed sedatives or another attempted medical intervention. Those who stretched hard drinking over years, like myself, landed in sanitariums. Sometimes for a long time, maybe permanently. Severe alcoholics were admonished and shoved aside. Those who didn't die were hidden in facilities for the insane. Until the 1930s, if your alcoholism reached levels considered chronic or acute, you were in serious trouble.

Alcoholics Anonymous developed in the second half of the 1930s, an off-shoot of the Bible-centric Oxford Group in the 1920s. Inter-weaving Bible lessons and then-contemporary life skills into *12 steps of action*, the book "Alcoholics Anonymous" – commonly called the "big book" of AA – was published in 1939. Started by an addiction-specialist physician and a salesman and middling bond trader, Alcoholics Anonymous the movement initiated with small gatherings in private homes in Akron, Ohio, and built out from there slowly. The primary goal of AA is to get other alcoholics involved with the program, with the ultimate being the last step, which basically says seek out and help other alcoholics and instruct them to do as you did. In a way, the salesman carried great influence in the formative years, and created this system which today we might liken to multi-level marketing. Only, without the financial incentives. Included in the last goal of AA, the 12th and final step, is to seek and secure more AA participants, to try to "carry this message to alcoholics, and to practice these principles in all our affairs."

Growth of AA was not immediate. It would take some promotional luck, with attention in big publications of the day, over years to build the organization into the 1950s. Then, AA leaders pulled off a public relations coup to get the American Medical Association to declare alcoholism a *disease*. In reality, use of the word "alcoholic" was not widespread until AA's book. It was well-established as the first attempt at a written program that people could follow for help overcoming booze. That a physician was involved in its formation helped greatly; doctors were tired of problem drinkers.

The big book is heavy on the spiritual side. Many steps are based on biblical values, like confession, forgiveness, and power of prayer. While the book's text states more than once that the program is not religious, but *spiritual*, the tome uses the word *God* or *Him* over 200 times. Hardly changed since 1939, the book goes an extra mile to suggest the alcoholic find a power greater than themselves, to surrender to and lean on for lasting sobriety. Surrendering your will and life over to this higher power is the thing of AA.

The program used its persistent lobbying to get the disease designation, which boosted its reputation nationally. Eventually big book sales grew noticeably. Yet, the organization strictly stuck with its nonprofit status, ultimately adopting a marketing approach of *attraction rather than promotion*. You won't see paid advertisements promoting AA, nor many people pumping it up publicly. It's a program designed to be run by alcoholics, to reach out and be available for others suffering the same malady. Quite honestly, my thought on AA is, it's an incredible program. Personally, I think it's more for newcomers or those maybe in the first years of sobriety. I have never bought into the lifetime of meetings and a must-have-a-sponsor concept. In this, I know I'm not alone. I have friends who sobered with AA, but remained sober even after no longer attending meetings or otherwise being involved.

Today, AA is the most relied-upon go-to for people to sober up (just as the younger Narcotics Anonymous serves drug addicts, with the 12 steps adapted). I have attended at least a thousand AA and NA meetings since 2009, with six sponsors to date. Add to that an unknown number of "service" positions with various groups, where I made coffee for meetings, or greeted people arriving. I've driven dozens of miles to reach new meetings, and much more. My time invested in trying to work the AA program is significant. Yet, over a dozen years I kept going to rehabs, all of which promoted AA at varying levels. I'll leave it at that.

While some AA is evident at most rehabs, few make it *the* entire program. What would be the point? Alcoholics Anonymous is free and optional.

Why go out of your way to secure a rehab bed, when you could get something any time free? A reason AA is not the primary framework for rehab programs is that it's not considered *medical treatment*, so insurance won't pay for it. (Some states actually forbid private centers from promoting AA or similar 12-step programs; I'll only assume it's a separation-of-church-and-state thing). So, few rehabs will host AA meetings *instead of groups*. Rehabs get paid for attendees in groups, but not for AA meetings. In fact, in Hawaii it's illegal for rehabs to include AA in structured programs. They will suggest and recommend AA or the steps, and let clients leave campus for meetings and all, but Hawaii rehabs cannot base programs on AA or its spinoffs.

Rehabs generate revenue in many ways. No surprise, a biggie is billing insurance. Insurers will pay for a client's monthly fee, plus sometimes extras like medications. Attendance in groups is routinely covered. As stated, new rehabbers will get used to meeting facilitators asking immediately about the sign-in sheet. "Everybody sign?" is sure to be heard. Signatures on sign-in sheets represent dollars. Daily, rehabbers will sign at least one sign-in sheet, and up to maybe six in a day, especially weekdays. Group sessions will have at least a dozen clients each. Do the math. Groups are profit centers.

What I don't get is when rehabs get a program assistant, or maybe someone else, even a volunteer, to host group sessions. Aren't groups covered by insurance due to *medical* benefits? Shouldn't groups be funded only if they are facilitated by someone trained or certificated to do so? How is a program assistant educated or trained to understand medical principles involved with treatment for addiction? Unless rehabs are billing and pretending their groups are run by certificated professionals. I doubt it. Yet, even with a volunteer hosting a group, we must sign. Signing becomes a Pavlovian thing – if rehabbers see a sign-in sheet laying on a table, chances are solid they will have an urge to seek a pen to sign it. Sometimes old sign-in sheets are left behind, and there might be two or more on a table without a group host in sight. In such instances I signed them all. Screw it. You can get in trouble for missing a group, they say.

Meetings by AA are not profitable. Still, rehabbers will hear plenty about those steps, and the need to get a sponsor. There is a good chance they will be required to attend, or asked to attend, 12-step meetings. My first rehabs were very heavy on the 12-step meetings. At AIA, it was a rare to have a night off. We'd even get vanned to a meeting on a Sunday, in a fire station of all places. Tarzana also had many, requiring the rearrangement of the big dining area nightly to get heavy round tables off to the side and the entire room filled with chairs lined up facing the same way. Meetings there would be open to outsiders and regularly seated many dozens, probably pushing 100 at times. Being allowed to commingle with visiting non-rehabbers with clean or sober time seemed beneficial; Redgate in Long Beach did this very well. Rehabs were plenty clear about rules for the comingling, and assigned plenty of staff to monitor.

I remember in TTC No. 2, I ended up serving as "meeting coordinator," the person responsible for the set-up and take-down of the dining room for each 12-step meeting. I was assigned the role apparently because I helped more than other clients when the previous guy was in charge, and constantly made recommendations on how to manage it better. It was like, *Okay wise guy, you do it.* My mouth, so often a troublemaker.

That was not an easy gig, getting volunteers to help pop heavy round tables on their sides, to roll to the rear against a wall. Then, using flat dollies to haul a hundred or so chairs from other rooms on campus into that dining area. Finally, after the meeting, returning all the chairs to other rooms, and re-setting the round tables for the next day's breakfast. For some reason they made us sign in to these meetings, which to me was curious because I assumed they couldn't bill for 12-step meetings, but maybe they did. Most likely it was just to monitor that we all were in attendance, and not sleeping or hiding in our rooms. Anyway, signing at the end created a hassle as everyone crowded around a single table to sign. It got in the way at a time when everyone was pooped, especially myself.

You get tired at night. Days are packed with groups or other activities like counselor meetings, and your eyes take a beating staring at whiteboards and printed materials, and lasting hours inside dry air-conditioned rooms. To have to then be active at night, especially in a physically and mentally challenging job like managing meetings, you get exhausted at the end. Which made me testy at times. Not good for recovery, for both myself, and whoever was the target of my wrath. I especially ragged on clients who never seemed to volunteer to help, or just stood around staring and got in the way. I'd give them shit about it verbally; sometimes they'd bark back. Honestly, no rehab should be forcing clients to do work so challenging that it causes stress. Tarzana does, though.

During my first TTC stint, I was laundry coordinator, overseeing a little room with eight huge stacked washer-dryers to serve 80 or so people. There was a schedule indicating days of the week for washing for batches of rooms, but many clients cheated, a reason a coordinator was necessary. The cheating was constant. When people forgot to move their clothes from washer to dryer, or left them in the dryer, it clogged the process and con-sumed a limited amount of time for clothes washing (say, 7 a.m. to 7 p.m.). A whiteboard was in the room where you were supposed to write your name and room number when you took a washer. This way, we could ensure only clients scheduled to use the room were doing so; and also to indicate who to track down for forgotten clothes batches. It was a bit more complicated than it might seem. I learned many adults arrive in rehab with no, or very limited, experience with laundry.

Everyone knows who's the laundry coordinator. Many clients asked for favors, like letting them know when there might be a gap when washers were free, or even doing really late loads. Ultimately staff warned me more than once that I had to lock the door at 7 p.m. no matter what. (Good rule, by the way, as the room had blind spots and an old unused shower where I'm sure night smoochings occurred). Left your clothes in there? Gotta wait 'til morning to get it, is what I had to say. I had a key, and people were constantly coming into my room while lights were out and I tried to sleep, begging me to open the laundry room which thankfully was not far away (a reason why I took the gig; also so I could do laundry whenever I wanted, a slick Rehab All-Star maneuver). Balancing staff's orders with being a nice helpful guy caused some stress. Not as much as years later managing night meetings, but still stress, which as stated is not good in early recovery. And even if I'd already been there a month or two, I was still in early recovery. Heck, we're all in *early recovery* the whole first year, probably longer.

Funny story about those meetings during TTC stay No. 1. The 12-step meetings were like 90 to 120 minutes long, with a 10-minute break in the middle. As with most rehab stays, I'd become an avid reader, almost to an excessive level. I'm also no fan of night meetings, something carried over from my news reporting and political aide days when I spent hours sitting through boring government meetings after sunset. Basically I'd been doing meetings multiple times every week for over two decades. For one housing project, as a consultant to the applicant I attended *at least* two dozen planning commission and city council meetings over two years. I remember monitoring the last games of baseball's American League Championship Series from my phone in October in *both* 2003 *and* 2004, when my Red Sox were good. (I'm still miffed at the City of Moorpark for that). I missed a lot due to those night meetings, and as I aged, I had enough. Night meetings are a burnout. Rarely would employers let you sleep in the next day to make up for it. My jobs were at-will; there was no overtime, and days could end up 12 or 14 hours long, followed by an early start the following day. It was unhealthy, and one of many things that contributed to my drinking volumes. I found it hard to wind down after meetings to get to sleep, worsening the situation.

Anyway, at TTC, in that hallway bathroom I mentioned with the three showers, there was one set aside for disabled persons which was bigger with a wooden bench that folded out from the wall. The showers had plastic curtains you could not see through, and the disabled shower happened to be next to the entrance door and would get blocked when the door was opened wide. It dawned on me: someone could sit in there, up on the wall seat with feet up and curtain closed, and be well-hidden.

So I developed a habit of not returning to the meeting for the second half. We'd hit the break, and I'd get into the shower and close the curtain, with a book, and sit on the fold-out seat with feet up. I'd read for many minutes, faintly hearing the goings-on of the meeting down the hall. People might sporadically come in, but they'd push the door open to block my stall, and they wouldn't fool around because they were expected to return to the meeting. I had no watch or phone to tell time, so I'd just listen for big chatter coming down the hall to know the meeting had ended, and it was time to blend back in with the clients. It worked many times.

Of course, I have a big mouth and told some roommates. So now and then, someone would step out of the second half of that meeting, enter the bathroom, and suddenly rip the curtain aside which would scare the shit out of me. Rule-breaking at TTC was serious, and could carry harsh consequences. I determined years later, the tough love bullshit is dated. In my opinion it was ineffective, and probably costly. I remember constant blow-ups and fights and program ejections at TTC. Way more than any other rehab, except maybe the Salvation Army which (at least in Long Beach) treated clients poorly. What I noticed was, at rehabs with fewer rules, and maybe also a bit more lenient with enforcement, there were fewer incidents. Less tantrums, fewer people getting ejected, not as many clients walking out, all of which *costs programs money*. It takes a lot of time and energy to intake rehab clients, and to keep proper records as they stay. I guess some rehabs figure it out, while others stick with what causes money-losing headaches.

* * *

I witnessed no "return visitors" at TTC No. 2 – no one like Josh returning to AIA. So, no rehab all-stars that I can remember at Tarzana. I did have a sponsor for my second TTC stay who ended up taking me with him to outside meetings. A client with me there in 2013, he sobered and was long-clean by 2018. Not an all-star, but a great guy and super example of rehabbing success, and still a contact on Facebook. I felt bad letting him down once I failed and disappeared in 2018.

Entering TTC the first time, I was told in advance that an old high school buddy was already inside. My source, the old friend who got me into TTC immediately, kind of broke the confidentiality rule most rehabs prefer due to medical privacy laws. Rehabs are considered hospital settings and therefore under privacy rules often referred to as HIPAA, for the Health Insurance Portability and Accountability Act enacted in 1996 to protect privacy and security of patient health information. I have been in sober living programs that were very cognizant of HIPAA requirements. Of course I don't blame my old school friend for this. Few "normies" are aware, and besides, I was grateful to get in TTC quickly.

Walking down the crowded hallway when I first arrived in residential, I saw the buddy, let's call him Chad, cruisin' by wearing his trucker ball cap. I called out his last name, and it took a few moments to register, but he finally recognized me. It had been many years, since I used to stop by his sandwich shop periodically (sometimes to buy small amounts of cocaine from an employee there, true story). He was fairly well-known in our hometown.

Chad had been at TTC for several months. He looked great, the same tanned, chilled good-lookin' surfer-type dude from school. I thought, *I never saw him smashed.* Never really knew he drank. I learned he ended up renting a small cottage in an unincorporated enclave of our hometown, and in the end rarely left the structure due to nonstop beer drinking. New rehabbers will hear similar stories. It usually precedes the "end," or period just before we realize treatment is required. For some of us, there's no debate. We drink ourselves out of usefulness and need help to continue living.

Chad explained the demise of his sandwich store franchise, due to opening a new shop in the north Valley. It shows the fragility of small businesses. He said one decision on a single new location doomed the franchise, which he'd built with his father with two locations in our hometown. I would probably drink over it, too.

I marveled how long he'd already been there, and Chad said he was in no hurry to get out, that he treated TTC as a long vacation, a getaway from the hurry-worry world. He was always calm, nothing seemed to bother him – the opposite of my anxious whining self. He just listened and observed. Chad was there long before I arrived, and stayed after I left. It would be five years, just before my return to TTC, that I would speak with him on the phone. His was among many calls I made trying to escape a horrific sober living house in Compton. At that time he was sympathetic, but like almost everyone else, unable to help. Compton was a terrible disaster still burned into my memory.

Chad luckily "got it" and didn't return. A mutual high school buddy of Chad and I, who got into TTC after us with help from the same source, didn't make it. I still see tribute Facebook posts on Stevie's birthday. Rehabbers, especially us return customers, will encounter deaths of people who were comrades in recovery or rehabs. I can't put a number on how many friends and close acquaintances I've lost. It's in the dozens, maybe 25, and probably more since we lose track of many after leaving rehab. Sometimes a death is surprising, but too often, not so much. Some rehabbers seem to just keep living regardless of relapses, refusing to quit. Some poor souls live on to suffer indefinitely.

See my 2017 chapter for details. There's an old medical study where they put a mouse into a cage with two options to drink from, one with water, the other laced with cocaine. The subjects would hit the tiny cocaine faucet and keep hitting it until they died. It was an early instance where scientists learned shortfalls in the brains of mammals. I know of humans who died like that in a way. I played the mouse several times and got lucky to break from the psychosis.

People entering their first rehab should know that some among you will die. It's important to acknowledge for a number of reasons, top among them being, if you don't take this rehab stuff seriously, we could be discussing *your death.* As Bob Mould sang in song, "If you don't stop and smell the roses now, they might end up on you." In early recovery it's a significant challenge to get past tragic events like the passing of someone you know. Even if you hardly knew the person, in reality when you hear of a recovery colleague's death, it conjures up memories of smiles or laughs that don't seem too far past. It also can bring regrets, that maybe you should have done more or could have been there for them. Remember what was stated in this book's Foreword. James said he wished he could have been there more.

My first experience with this was the Washington state trucker who months after being with me in my first rehab house shot himself. He was very quiet and showed no hints of suicidal consideration. At the Salvation Army, a fellow a few years older died not long after leaving the Sally of sleep apnea, which he suffered through for six months at the facility. I remember hearing his tremendous snores through a wall each night. Another who was with me both Sally stays was found dead on the side of a random stranger's house in South Bay. We rarely get details, most certainly no autopsy confirmations. Sometimes it's not the addiction itself that kills; it's the tendency of the afflicted to *ignore health care* or going to see doctors. Very poor health can go unnoticed if poisons keep you numb all hours of the day. Toss in unsanitary situations, like sleeping on concrete or in bushes, and it's a recipe for illness.

These were guys I spent a lot of time with not long prior. These deaths did not make me relapse, but they sure hit hard. I can just envision AA old-timers saying, "I stayed sober through the death of my spouse!" Well, good for you. For most in the first months or years of recovery, it's difficult to get past. Swift emotional shifts mess you up. Rack up a bunch over a short period of time, and the likeliness of relapse increases. Remember this last part, because much of this book is about how to do things to *increase the odds* of staying clean and sober.

It's vital for at least two reasons. First, the odds are stacked tremendously against the afflicted. Remember the success rate for AA, meaning people who stayed sober the rest of their lives due to program participation, is about 7%, give or take some percentage points. Avid AA members might argue it's 10%, some might say it's like 25%, maybe even a bit higher. Whatever, it can't be even half, so the odds are not good. Recovering fully for life is very hard. The odds for success are not great to begin with. The most rehabbers can do is take actions to *better those odds*; or avoid anything that might *reduce the odds*.

Like hitting Las Vegas with teen-agers for a holiday weekend punk rock festival with just 75 days sober. Be very wary of these choices. That skill, to know what to avoid no matter what, is among the very top you can develop for recovery. For things you cannot avoid, be sure to have tactics developed. Start nurturing coping skills right away, by attending 12-step meetings consistently, or doing something daily to nurture your recovery. Anything. A whole bunch of little things, like staying in contact with others in recovery, or just talking with clean and sober people, or remembering spiritual breaks during the day, can help increase success rates. Work to improve and maintain your recovery daily, and you might not have to be a Rehab All-Star.

* * *

Memories from the first TTC stay include pink-slipping my truck to my son before I went in, with the cocky attitude that I would just buy another car once sober. (It never happened by the way, and he's still driving the truck in Missouri 12 years later). That short drive from Simi Valley to Tarzana was painful, with Dad in his truck. By this time he had to be sick of driving to rehabs – and at that moment was unaware he'd do it again. Dad was a trooper and an angel. Mom at one point was so frustrated she told Dad that she wished I'd never been born. The addiction turned me into a devil child.

At AIA during intake they search property bags thoroughly. At TTC they did the same, plus a full strip search. Even when down to just my underwear briefs, they asked if I had any patches underneath. I said I didn't know what they were talking about. Stick patches to get high? Weird. Must be a Valley thing, I thought.

This rehab was filled with gang-bangers, wannabe gangsters, lost causes, and junkies, some of them not all that bright. One roommate had his phone ring in his pocket *while* he was talking with a high-level supervisor in a hallway. Having a mobile phone inside was a no-no. Not knowing to turn the sound off was a no-no-no way.

We had van rides to meetings, just not near as many as at AIA. I had a visitor, a friend from girls softball and fellow Red Sox fan, Mike E., which was way cool. Eventually my new girlfriend began visiting every week. I was constantly on the hunt for quarters to make nightly calls. She attended a Halloween party there, even getting me a yellow shirt with a black zig-zag across it horizontally so I could be Charlie Brown with my shaved big head. Charlie Brown with a goatee was the joke; she dressed as Lucy, and it was a bit weird dancing sober in that dining room. For me, dancing was a smashed-drunk occasion. I would get passes and go have sex in her car in daylight. Once I even snuck out at night to do this, then creeped back in through an open kitchen door. Recovery was just not the first priority. No wonder I kept being a return customer.

Perhaps there were just too many characters, and innumerable entertainment opportunities. One was a little guy in the bed above me, a meth addict from Arkansas missing his front four teeth. One time he got a pass to visit a dentist for new teeth, and since he was new, the program assigned a mentor to accompany him, which was lucky me. His girlfriend picked us up, and somewhere in Pasadena they got into an argument, and toothless man threatened to kick out the front windshield if she didn't stop the car. She stopped, and he got out and ran away mid-intersection. So there I was, in the back seat with a stranger and no phone and no idea what to do regarding the rehab. It wasn't like I could find a pay phone and say, *Hey, sorry, but I lost the guy.* Luckily he returned quickly and we made it to the dentist, and back in a reasonable amount of time. Still, he sure was a hothead.

Eventually he was assigned nightly cleanings of that big hall bathroom we shared with the general population, with the big disabled stall for my hidden reading. Well, my bunkmate would return at night after cleaning that thing, with stories galore, mostly bitching on and on. The whining became routine, and it triggered an idea. The next time I went into a stall to take a dump, I pulled off little pieces of toilet paper and chewed them to make mushy little balls, then threw them against a stall wall where they would stick. I hit the two plastic dividers, then the door, then for good measure chewed up two more and tossed them straight up to stick *on the ceiling.* Then I left, and quietly waited.

Every morning we had an all-clients meeting on the patio where the student council president would say something and announce passes (and mentors) for the day and what not. At the end of his spiel, the leader asked if anyone had anything to share with the "family." Toothless man stood up and, in his awesome Southern drawl, said, "You know, I clean that big hall bathroom, and I ask if you could please clean after yourself. I mean, I went in there last night, and someone threw *spitballs* all over. I mean, *spitballs. Who does shit like that?*"

I was sitting next to Chad about as far away from that dude as we could get, and it was the hardest effort ever to refrain from bursting out laughing. Painfully hard. A few other family members spoke after, but every time I'd peek over at bathroom cleaner's scowling red face, I would start convulsing to hold back chuckles, like holding back killer hiccups. Damn that was hard. And I knew he was a hothead so it was imperative to keep it together. I wonder if the spitballs are still on the ceiling.

Not long after that, the student council leader got drunk on a pass, returned to campus, and punched a client who worked the commissary. The punch victim ended up being my sponsor five years later. After the incident he was called Shiner by a dude who hosted a weekly meeting in Woodland Hills we frequented, who apparently made a lot of money playing keyboards for Fleetwood Mac. My future sponsor for a while had a black eye, always a comic point in AA meetings. (Once I arrived at Aloha House with two black eyes; they called me Raccoon). They ejected the student council leader, which was eye-opening. I mean, a top client, someone given respect and expected to serve as an exemplary example of recovery, went out and got drunk. Then came back and punched someone. What the heck?

Not long after another client, who rumor had it was somehow related to the rehab's owner, returned one night smashed drunk trying to sneak in a 12-pack of beer. He was not ejected, and I was amazed how he walked around afterward pretending nothing happened. Not long after that, a roommate we called Rooster went screaming down the hall carrying all his clothes in a stuffed green trash bag, yelling all the way out the back gate to who knows where. I started getting accustomed to such incidents and outbursts, which would have been foreign at AIA.

* * *

My **TTC No. 2** stay lasted from July 31 to mid-October 2018. For both stays I was not provided an exit date, nor in reality even an exit plan. Maybe some general discussion about what I should do, but I don't remember anything concrete. The counselors were unremarkable. One was sleepy most times from side work as an overnight security guard. The area was not cheap to live in, and most rehabs don't pay well. The 2018 visit was a zoo experience. I still don't know how they fit so many souls in there. That second counselor was green and learning. Not a bad guy, just in way over his head.

They say there are over 134,000 substance abuse counselors in the United States, maybe as high as 483,500 if you count behavioral disorder therapists, mental health counselors, specialized physicians, or others whose work is related to addiction. In my journey, I've tapped all of the above. It's probably still not enough trained professionals compared with the frightening number of alcoholics and addicts.

At TTC, I learned there are worse rehabs than AIA. What I did not know was, TTC would *not be my worst rehab experience.* That would encompass almost all of 2015, and a good chunk of 2016. In between, 2014 was a rare year of no rehabs. Looking back, I realized my no-rehab years tended to be worse than those filled with rehab time.

CHAPTER 4

SALVATION ARMY
2015 AND 2016

Redemption?

A girlfriend yanked me from TTC No. 1 in early November 2013, and we lived together in her garage-converted apartment in our hometown until the end of 2014. That was my first break from the nearly constant rehabs of 2012 and 2013. And it was a rough 13-plus months, maybe my toughest stint to that point, saved only by an angel I met by chance playing an app game on an iPhone.

I admit, we had some fun. In the past I was probably a hedonist when freed from constraints of marriage, family, career, or structure. But all told, 2014 was a disaster. She was an alcoholic not putting much effort into avoiding the poisons, and I didn't last long. Within weeks of exiting TTC, she was arrested on suspicion of felony assault, a few days before Thanksgiving. Assault on me, right off the bat, there in the apartment. That was a sign of what was to come the following months.

We'd been drinking, as usual, and apparently I did something to really set her off, and she punched my face three times. Good times. Unfortunately for her, I called the cops, and a ring on her finger broke the skin a little right next to my mustache, and off to jail she went. I woke the next day in a hotel room not far away, hardly a memory of what happened. Basically the police treated me as they do female domestic violence victims, getting me to a hotel room to get away from the property. I'm unaware how it was funded.

Months later, she would pick me up exiting jail in Ventura, where she had me sent after yet another drunken dispute. The timing worked out well for her. She waited for me to walk out of jail so I could testify in court that morning, just across a courtyard, *for her case*. They had postponed her first hearing, and seeing I was already next door in Ventura for the second hearing, she picked me up so I could ask the judge to drop the felony charge. So there I was, sitting next to the person who had just put me in jail, wearing the same clothes from hours in a cell, in court *next to someone charged with assaulting me*, waiting to beg for forgiveness to a judge. Pretty much because I had to, since the suspect was after all my landlord. Who else on Earth can say that? Ultimately there was no charge. The county just lost the case. That shit never happens to me, but it did for my girlfriend-landlord.

That year, I was arrested at least six times for public intoxication, usually right in front of our apartment, on a lengthy driveway right off Alamo Street. We lived in a semi-rural zone, where chickens ran wild on properties around us. Though I probably could have run to elude the coming police, the distance from our front door to the street must have seemed daunting since I always just waited to be taken away. You could literally see the police station from our property. She never got over the $2,000 it cost for her arrest, to bail out fast because she couldn't get along with cellmates. She got mouthy to gang-banger chicks, then had to get out pronto. That was my fault somehow. Eventually the cops warned that they were being called to the address too much, and they would bill the property owner for any more calls. That seemed to calm things down. However, the bail money animosity sizzled.

I didn't work much that year. The first few months I had a decent contract with an online education company focused on selling insect kits to teachers, but I relapsed out. I had another job that summer, after moving in with my folks for a spell, at a website marketing company in Woodland Hills, but I drank myself out of that (and out of my parents' place, too). In September, laying on grass near City Hall, homeless and partially drunk, a friend from Moorpark called to ask for public relations help in a battle with his landlord, a monopolistic public utility. That job was needed and quite timely and got me back into our apartment. Then I was laid off before Thanksgiving, and then again just before Christmas, by the same friend. That year sucked.

By December, both of us sensed the end. I was let go the second time, and having no income made the home environment worse. The future for work and home life seemed bleak, and I didn't have any ideas or leads to get out. Around this time both of us were playing a Scrabble-like game app off phones, in which you make words for points, but it also allowed messaging with opponents. Words with Friends used locations to match people geographically for contests. Randomly I was matched with a pretty blond whose WWF profile photo showed her smiling big in a bright blue Los Angeles Dodgers tee. I messaged and learned she lived in Fillmore, about a 45-minute drive north of Simi Valley in Ventura County. She was good at Scrabble, and quite smart. We had graduated CSUN the same period, and both were former athletes. How we developed all the back-and-forth banter remains a mystery, but in total, this new friend served as a counselor, shrink, and mentor all in one package.

Over time she became a great friend, sometimes prophetic in her predictions regarding my recovery, someone who always said what needed to be said. No coddling, that's for damn sure. I probably leaned on Shannon because I wasn't being intellectually stimulated at home, and without the release of a workplace I had little human contact. With no car, I relied on who I lived with to get around, and did not have much alone time. I did not hang out with friends. Rarely did I take her with me to friends' events, mainly because I was not being invited. Admittedly, that was at least partially because of my affliction. I closed most everyone off. I was isolating, albeit with one other person, to drink and smoke pot. Just a lost soul who recently had his wife, family, home, and way of life disappear.

One afternoon returning from work or a store run, my girlfriend decided to tell me she met someone on WWF, ironically from Fillmore, and that he visited and they had a little foreplay on the couch. It ended quickly and nothing more was to come of it, she said, insisting she wanted to be up front with me. Honestly, looking back, it was an opportunity for her to begin to shoo me away. Thankfully, it worked. It planted a seed in my mind: *How can things possibly get any worse?*

Christmas approached. My relationship with Shannon grew seemingly by the hour, all through Words with Friends. I reported everything happening at home, all about my alcoholism and recovery efforts, and Shannon did not hold back. I'd pop a word onto the game table, then report about the latest drunken situation. She'd set a word and respond. This went on for a while.

The girlfriend took us to my parents' home for Christmas, and it turned out to be the last time I was with my brother and his kids, my niece and nephew. It was December 2014. There's a photo somewhere on social media capturing the occasion. I may have cropped out the girlfriend.

A couple days after Christmas, Shannon and I arranged to meet. She had landed a job unbelievably close by, a short walk from my apartment, at an animal medical clinic in Simi. She said she liked dive bars, and one of my favorites was around the corner. We met, sipped Bass beers, and played darts. She showed a hell of a throwing arm, chucking darts like baseballs kind of side-armed from about 10 feet away. It was funny, but I got a tad nervous at the velocity of the darts and how they punished the board on impact. Patrons noticed, haha. On the jukebox, playing was the beginning of the Rush album "2112," which we had chatted about just days before. It was surreal; the song is not a hit single or something normally found on a jukebox.

Through all our messages, I told Shannon my entire recovery story, and she consoled, asked a lot of questions, and advised me to escape and pursue the life she felt was meant for me. She once said, "You need to get sober so you can help other people get sober." Still valid.

Upon leaving the bar, due to the beers, she decided to skip the long and winding drive to Fillmore and stay the night in a hotel in central Simi. I joined, and never returned to that little apartment and that girlfriend again. I chose to be homeless rather than return. I can't entirely blame the girlfriend. I was just not in a healthy state of mind. I visited a final time a few days later to retrieve clothes and property. I wasn't invited inside.

It was instant homelessness, and I did not anticipate the impact. Walking out of that apartment would be the first step toward getting out of my hometown of 37 years, changing my life. I am unsure I would have survived had I stayed in Simi Valley, not because of the town or people there, but because I did not comprehend the severity of my sickness. I did not yet have the knowledge and tools to get better there. Staying would mean repeating the year over and over.

Shannon was kind and gave me a couple of days on her living room couch in Fillmore, even though she had a teenage daughter with her there. I detoxed badly with the shakes, which I think shocked her. She worked with me to craft an email to my mother, explaining that this angel took me in, and that I needed help to move forward with living arrangements after my escape from the apartment. Mom responded that they would buy me a week's hotel stay in Simi, to allow time to get my shit together. My parents did that more than once, and I never got my shit together in a week. Soon I was again on the streets, albeit staying sober and in touch with Shannon. With every hotel week from my parents, I just partied my ass off, but that time I was good because Shannon would visit almost every night before commuting home. Our talks helped a lot to calm my nerves.

Eventually I found a bike locker next to a courthouse that was hardly used. It was a hexagon design, with each locker shaped like a slice of pizza, the door being the widest part. It was about rib-cage tall, and each slice could fit a bike, plus a little extra space if you were clever. I took one to store my bike and clothes, and another to sleep in, head-first, feet at the door. I'm not making this up: in the middle of winter in a cold desert evening climate, I spent nights sleeping in a bike locker. The door was not solid, with slats to vent, so the fog and cold crept in. Texting Shannon every night, we were kind of a semi-couple for that very brief period. There was a homeless shelter program in town where sleeping arrangements rotated among churches, so you had to know the schedule and where to go each evening, and be sober.

Shannon could not house me due to work and the daughter, and I understood. I was still for the most part a stranger, with a substance use problem at that. I promised to remain sober and stay in touch, and we had a little verbal agreement that if I could stay sober and get my shit together, we *just might* date. I think the agreement was to be sober for a year and then talk. A challenge, but a nice incentive.

I adored Shannon, and being with her was like a dream. I lasted 30 days. Eventually my addiction wholly took over. Looking back, it was kind of a good thing. Though I hadn't drank in days, I still needed significant treatment for whatever ailed my brain. Doing the cold turkey thing on the streets could only last so long. I needed help that would stick long-term. I was going it alone to get to 30 days. It couldn't have lasted.

It was Super Bowl Sunday, and as with all relapses, for an unknown reason I decided it was a good idea to drink, and watched the game at a nearby bar. Where the money came from, who knows? I watched the first half then drank too much, and slithered back to my bike locker since hitting a church shelter was out because they tested breaths for alcohol to enter. The next morning, Shannon texted to congratulate me for 30 days sober. That milestone happened to be that day. I was honest and admitted I'd slipped, and her reaction was not hesitant. She messaged that she was devastated and that was that. The last time I saw her in person was a few days later when she dropped off clothing I'd left at her house. The last we touched, I patted pieces of leaves and grass from her rear end since we had sat on the ground to talk a little. "You just wanted to touch my butt," was one of the last things she said, in a classic Shannon smart-alecky way.

Shannon ended up getting a boyfriend soon thereafter and it wasn't long before they married. I discovered this while in the next rehab, and was quite distressed about it. She had blocked me on social media, so all I could see were her profile photos, which were of her and the future husband, as if a message that she'd moved on for good. Well, she had. Somehow months later we reconnected, probably after I sent multiple requests. For some reason she finally relented, and we remain friends to this day. She moved to southern Nevada not far from Las Vegas. Over a decade, she would experience many of my epic relapses, noticed mainly because of my total disappearance on Facebook, many times scaring the bejeezus out of her. She and many others would connect on Facebook looking for me, some believing me dead. This happened more than I like to admit. She always reconnected, and admonished me *fiercely* each time. At least once she threatened to disappear, but she never did. A true gift from the Spirit of the Universe, for which I remain grateful.

* * *

A decades-long run living in Simi Valley ended in February 2015. I struggled badly living on the streets, finding nooks at closed government offices or nearby to sleep in the cold since I couldn't avoid the booze to sleep in a shelter. I honestly don't remember much for a period of about three weeks. Except that a courthouse security guard caught onto the bike locker living and gave me a day to clear out and not return. That would cause a big problem; I had a bike and a tall plastic garbage can full of clothes. I had no options and walked away thinking I would just leave it all and let them toss it.

That night was one of the coldest I ever spent, with nothing but jeans and a denim jacket to keep warm, and a backpack for a pillow, in front of a shuttered book store across the street from the police station. It was maybe a football field's distance from my old apartment. I remember the foggy evening vividly. I crossed Alamo Street three times to visit an all-night convenience store, just to raise my body temperature temporarily. It was that cold. The second visit, the clerk forced me to buy a coffee, which I did before settling down to attempt to sleep again. The last visit, the clerk threatened to call the police.

The next morning, somehow I had change for a couple of airplane bottle shots of vodka, before hopping onto a bus destined for the other end of town several miles away, for breakfast and a shower at a nonprofit drop-in center for the needy. I ate, then used the bathroom for a shower and to shave my head, because you learn on the streets to *not look homeless*. You still had to get into stores and such, and to talk with officials who just might help you out. Beards and shaggy hair are telltale signs of homelessness.

Exiting the bathroom, someone said the executive director of the organization wanted to see me. Not all that long before, I did public relations work for them pro bono. I was known in the community for my writing and media abilities, and for doing work without fees. She pulled me aside. "We have been watching you for two weeks now, and you're going to die," she said. "You look terrible. We arranged for a bed for you at a rehab in Long Beach. We'll give you a ride. You have to be here tomorrow morning by 9, or don't ever come back." That last part was the kicker. Without their services, I'd be in serious trouble, and knew it.

I got help from my parents, for a night at their house. Dad visited me at the bike locker to retrieve my belongings, and the next morning he took me to the Samaritan Center. From there, the ride to Long Beach was a challenge, since the driver talked a lot about my need for God. I got some temporary relief, but the old rehab-ride anxiety overwhelmed. *Salvation Army?* What is *that?* I asked the driver, who explained a little, particularly the spiritual component. At that moment it didn't sound bad. I knew I was in trouble and needed a healthy heaping of help. I was very relieved to get off the streets; just the thought of a bed was attractive.

During a lengthy intake process, thank goodness the driver stuck around. I was rejected, because I had forgotten about snorting meth with a stranger in a hotel room a few nights prior. Meth usually exits the body in about 48 hours, but this time it stuck longer. I have vague memories of that hotel night doing meth. Scary.

At the start of the long ride back to Simi Valley, the driver pulled over and had me call my parents since she was unavailable to drive the next day. They were absolutely pissed but agreed that Dad would drive me back. After a night of drinking a lot of water, the next morning we arrived, I passed the pee test, and watched Dad walk out. It was Feb. 25, 2015. Dad would revisit once, many months later, with my youngest daughter. It would not be until Christmas that I would see my mother again. And that would be a somber reunion.

* * *

My hair was chopped down to nubble, and chin hair shaved, but they let the mustache remain. I was allowed to choose a new wardrobe from the Army's adjacent thrift store. I was assigned to a room with three beds and three tall metal lockers unattached to the walls. Against the wall to the left when you entered was a young, taller, well-built, and mass-tattooed white kid who would make life exciting a few weeks later. The first morning was mayhem. Early wake-up call, rush to make my bed as directed by roommates, a long line into breakfast for a huge plate of food. Stuffed, then more rushing to a large room with moveable seats, for a brief chapel service and encouragement. This is how we kicked off each work day. Which was every day except Sundays, when we had to attend a formal chapel service that wouldn't get us back home until after noon. We never had a full day off.

Weekdays after the brief morning chapel, we were marched to work, in a huge adjacent warehouse. It was 6:30 a.m. We would work in a dusty, sweaty setting until 3:30 p.m. We would get a 30-minute lunch, plus two 15-minute breaks in a small enclosed asphalted patio area. Sometimes they'd have coffee, snacks, or juices for us.

As a beneficiary (that's what they call clients, I am not making this up), the first month at the Sally you cannot leave the property after work. Perhaps the best aspect of the Salvation Army's Adult Rehabilitation Center (ARC) in Long Beach was the freedom to sign out, leave the property, and go out into the community when not working or otherwise ordered. As long as we'd been there 30 days and behaved. They used an interesting form of the caste system, where you were identified by the color of your lanyard strap holding your required-at-all-times ID badge. If you just started, you wore a red string, meaning no privileges. Barely above that was a yellow rope, which is for troublemakers. Break a rule, and wear yellow for a week or two (or, in my case for one infraction, three weeks). Green ropes let you leave after work to see the town, hit the library for internet access, or general mischief. As with almost all rehabs, upon entry they took our mobile phones, separating us from the world. Getting online at the library as much as possible became imperative. Especially if you had fantasy sports teams to manage.

Other than getting out of the huge, very old, dry facility, life there was miserable. To top it off, it was a *six month* program. It took a while for that to register. My first few days hanging clothes for hours in a dust-choked warehouse, it began wearing on me. My thoughts raced. *Could I possibly last here?* I had graduated from 28 days to two or three months, to half a year in rehab. Think about that progression, over a short period of time. It should have been a sign that my illness was ramping up.

I would stay there for 10 months.

* * *

I grabbed clothes off a plastic table, weaved a hanger into each article, and hung each piece on a thick horizontal metal pole about eye level. These garments, donated from people in that region of Los Angeles, from the Orange County line deep into Torrance and the Palos Verdes Peninsula, would be dumped in batches at the end of a row of tables where *beneficiaries* one at a time grabbed items and hung them. The racks held 25 garments, at which point we would yell "Runner!" and a poor sap with that job would appear to replace your full rack with a fresh rack full of empty hangers. He then would take the full rack to someone somewhere back there to attach price tags with a plastic hand gun. It was a hella operation moving tons of material, and that was *just for clothing*. There were many other departments, from books to shoes to electrical and more. Downstairs, refrigerators, furniture, and mattresses arrived and departed constantly.

In the clothing department, the start point for newcomers, about a dozen of us would stand on either side of the plastic tables, and those runner guys would pile clothes onto one end. Then we'd grab garments, and scoot the pile along the line to reach each bennie who grabbed articles to hang. You grabbed a blouse, for instance, and a hanger that came with the fresh rack, and hung the blouse onto that same rack. Then repeat, ad nauseum. No talking. At the end of the plastic tables was a conveyor belt. Items damaged, or that we couldn't sell in stores like socks, underwear, or anything overly sexy, were carried to a huge hole in the concrete and dumped into a big pile downstairs to be squished into a cube and shipped to China for pennies on the pound. They worked hard to monetize pretty much everything that came in.

For that, they dedicated extraordinary amounts of energy. We'd get some donations from nearby, but the operation mostly depended on reaching outside Long Beach to get tractor-trailer trucks full of donated crap daily. Multiple trucks would head out early each morning and visit homes, often of the deceased when survivors didn't want to deal with all the "stuff." Basically anyone who called asking for pickup of unwanted items. The flow of donations into this facility was mind-boggling. It was a never-ending battle for us bennies to get whipped (figuratively, of course, though I bet some supervisors considered it) into working harder and faster by uppity warehouse staff. I remember during the first hours thinking to myself, "*This is bad.* Is this what to expect *every day?*" Or, to quote a friend from my hometown, "When you wake up in jail, you think, 'I'm a *baaad* boy.'" That's how I felt, that I had truly reached rock bottom and was being punished. That, on the first day of work.

It *was* rock bottom. I wasn't in Arrowhead, for sure. Not even at TTC. These ARCs are all over the country, even in Hawaii, in Honolulu I learned. They are **not** substance abuse disorder *treatment* operations, so inclusion in this book may be unfair. They are designed to give destitute adults skills and habits to help them move on to become productive and self-reliant human beings. This all harkens back to why the Army was created, by some dude in

Britain in the 19th century when he noticed the destitute all over city streets and arranged a program to help them, hopefully cleaning up the streets in the process. With work and tough love, a strategy carried forward some 150 years, helping to get an innumerable number of souls into living situations. The goal was admirable; it's the modern management and execution that needs attention. Greed oozed from the institution, and I did not encounter much empathy from staff. Whatever the opposite of empathy is, most personnel there had it.

This doesn't mean there was no attempt to help us stay clean and sober. They required us to carry a little paper slip each week to gather signatures from hosts at 12-step meetings, to prove attendance at a mandatory five a week. So, after being brow-beaten in a dusty warehouse for hours, you usually had to walk or hitch a ride to a meeting to get your little paper card filled. Every week. On this, I was pretty good, but cheating was widespread. In fact, I noticed more shenanigans at the ARC than any other rehab, which is amusing since it had the strictest rules and enforcement.

You were assigned a counselor to meet with weekly, required to get a sponsor, and subject to random urine analyses tests, though not often. In a way it resembled a rehab. However, emphasized much more was Jesus, and working. The Sally is recognized as a Christian religion, same as Latter-Day Saints, episcopals, etc., and the ARC program is heavy on chapel twice a week, and little things biblically forbidden like swearing or spitting or anything sexual or sexually related. Unsure if that includes farting, though a colleague tested it to the extreme. I can't say I'd ever heard anyone threatened with punishment for rancid flatulence (George Church, RIP).

When they let us peruse the thrift store for our clothes, they required us to pick out a dress jacket, slacks, two dress shirts, and a tie for chapel Wednesday afternoons on site, and Sunday mornings off-site at a chapel for what is called the Corps. I'm still not clear exactly what the Corps is, but based on my observations it does tremendous work helping families and kids and the needy, providing food and clothes, religious services, and more. Years later I would attend a blended AA-Bible meeting at a Corps building on Maui.

The Corps was completely separate from our ARC. It seemed much of the operation has not changed much since the days of the English do-gooder who started it. As a journalist, I found some details and history interesting, even amusing. While there, I took advantage of the biggest book library of any rehab, and found some classics I always wanted to digest, like "Grapes of Wrath" by John Steinbeck. Interestingly, toward the end of the book, when the protagonist's family is trying to survive in California's Central Valley, the mother talks about her destitute husband. She said, "The Salvation Army made him crawl for his meals." This was written in the early 1930s! Fast-forward some 80 years, and there I was, not necessarily crawling, but sweating profusely every day for meals and a bed.

There is a tremendous amount of repetitiveness, so you have to some-how train your mind to endure. At least I did. Mental survival tactics applied by other inmates are unknown. You're always among males, most of them younger with the annoying habits of 20-somethings. Chicks and drugs were the hot topics for conversation, even though the Sally forbade it. My go-to was punk rock, and I found a few disciples, some who remain friends today. One beneficiary once worked at a Long Beach restaurant owned by the former drummer of Social Distortion, which caught my attention. A few years later while in a sober phase, Richard drove me to Social D's 40th anniversary show in Orange County. He also once drove me to Hollywood for an event honoring Johnny Ramone, at a historic cemetery where we visited the graves of both Johnny and Dee Dee Ramone of the Ramones.

I've been listening to punk rock since the mid-1980s. Having grown up with the greatest classic rock, due to a father in love with Elvis, the Stones, Beatles, Byrds, the Doors, and more, I was way into rock music. For some reason in my early college years, when I morphed into a rebel without a clue, I got dragged into punk rock starting with softball teammate James Swanson from Eagle Rock. We met at a ball diamond in the west Valley and are punk fanatics to this day. (In 2024 to 2025 I helped edit his book that was published, "Super Stoked," about how he grew his business with a healthy helping of punk rock principles). I go through phases where I am totally enamored with a single band, usually for years. Up to the ARC, it had been Social Distortion for probably a decade. When sober, I listen to punk rock constantly.

One of my favorite bands was Rancid out of the Bay Area, whose first radio hit was a song called "Salvation." The tune had a killer chorus where the backing singers barked in unison, "I want your salvation," after the lead singer asked a lady to show him what she had to give away. It's a groovy song with a killer chorus. Sounded great on the radio, though through 2015 I had not purchased any Rancid records. That would change.

One day, a few months into the Sally drudgery, we were working in the warehouse where I'd been assigned to a department called Bric-a-Brac. It turns out that hanging clothes is for beginners, or for troublemakers demoted to demeaning clothes hanging. It took maybe a week before I was promoted to a very fast-paced department where we sorted junk and knick-knacks all day. I started by pulling big full carts on wheels over to a big square wood table, then emptying all the contents for two co-workers to sort through all the shit to decide what could be sold and what would be tossed. Between them was a conveyor belt leading to an employee who hurriedly stuck price stickers on items the sorters had placed on the belt because they were clean and could sell. That was the main gist of the operation, getting items priced to fill blue plastic boxes that could be shipped to four stores our operation supported. All this energy was to ensure those stores were always fully stocked. A never-ending proposition.

After barely surviving a month or so of loading, I got a chance to be a sorter, which was cool because at my age the loading was physically demanding. Looking back, I don't know how I survived without blowing an anger fuse. I'd get cuts on my hands and fingers and bruises galore wrestling with heavy items in those rolling red carts, and was yelled at constantly to hurry up. It sucked.

Sorting, you just grabbed items on the table and chose one of three destinations for each. The best items were placed on the conveyor belt for pricing. Clothes or items for other departments (like shoes, books, or electrical) were tossed into flat bins off to the side, for transport elsewhere in the warehouse for others to deal with. A lot of stuff, I'll estimate at least a third if not half, was trashed. Finally, there was this big chain-link cage on wheels, like eight feet squared, where we would toss anything else. These were auction carts. Items tossed inside could be broken or damaged, or just things we couldn't sell in stores, but still were maybe desirable for someone out there. For instance, sex-related shit we always tossed into the auction cage. After we showed everyone and joked about it, of course. That poor middle-aged pricer woman working there every day among us juvenile-brained bennies.

Auction carts would get full and we'd call a runner to come roll it away, to be replaced with a fresh empty one. We would fill like a dozen a day – just a shitload of junk. Full carts were wheeled outside to be auctioned off on the warehouse yard, as a single bulk item, everything as-is. I was told dudes with pickup trucks would visit every weekday to bid cash to fill their trucks for transport to Mexico. Again, everything was monetized. I'm surprised they didn't figure out how to generate electricity from our movement at all times. Periodically the tall grouchy assistant warehouse supervisor would switch it up and I got brief stints as a runner – a guy who ran around and emptied full bins, and basically made sure nothing including trash got overwhelmed to slow the progress of processing junk. This was imperative, since tons of new junk came in every day. There were stacks of blue plastic boxes waiting for us to fill. We'd never catch up. We could only work our asses off to ensure we did not run out of space in the warehouse to allow more shit to come in.

Being a runner is just a step above being a loader. It was hard work, it just didn't involve being stuck in one spot lifting and dropping shit onto a table all day. One day as a runner, trying to keep my mind occupied during tedious work, the tune "Salvation" by Rancid popped into my head. For no reason, really. As I worked, in my mind I found myself singing along to the tune, especially the repeated chorus, "I want your salvation! Whoaaa-ooh." I hummed it a while, then it hit me. Wait a minute. *What is this song about?*

The shift mercifully ended, and I ran to my room, changed into clean clothes, then ran downstairs to sign out and get to the library. On a computer I Googled "Salvation" and Rancid, and landed on a Wikipedia page for the band. Sure enough, *the song was about the Salvation Army.* Not just the Salvation Army, but about its ARC! Specifically, the tune is about the band's leader and his experience working … in an ARC for six months while sobering up before forming Rancid! Just years after surviving the Sally, Tim Armstrong was getting famous on MTV.

It all made sense. The lyrics are not critical of the program, per se, but about Armstrong's perception of the donated items they handled. It sounds like he was a truck helper, one of the bennies assigned to team with a truck driver to help load and unload donations all day. Back-breaking work that I never did. While doing this, Armstrong noticed people lived extravagantly, with huge refrigerators and diamond rings and more, all these valuable items that they could afford to just give away. "I can't believe these people live like kings," is a memorable line.

That's the essence of our ARC work: collect, sort, and price a great variety of donated items to supply the adjacent thrift store, and also stores in Torrance, Downey, and Compton. The Torrance store in particular was of great importance, as it accepted donated items from affluent areas like the entire Palisades Peninsula, an affluent enclave between San Pedro and Torrance. The Torrance store was very big, and busy.

After working a full 44 hours a week, us newcomers had to do what I learned later was a no-no for ARCs. We were van-transported to a store to work a Saturday afternoon. Usually arranged in the classic caste system where we were forced to wear bright yellow vests. Might as well have put protective helmets on us, too, maybe even flags on sticks. Working the stores was no joke, being on your feet for another four hours (or more) after 44 hours of warehouse labor over six days. In stores we moved items around, were harassed by store managers stressed from being harassed by their bosses whoever they were. The whole operation seemed chock full of harassment, threats, and greed. I'd have sympathy for those store managers, but they were weasels or full-on assholes, especially at Torrance. While I only had to do that a handful of times, I found plenty of ways to screw off. It just felt like a way to send an FU to those managers and the Salvation Army.

I'd hide behind or even *inside* big furniture items, or find Bric-a-Brac junk to play with. One time after helping a couple fit a big bed into a pickup truck, I was tipped $20. Actually, they were tipping me and an employee whose job back there was loading purchased items into pickup trucks, or unloading donations, but he didn't see the exchange. Fuck him, I was broke, and in desperate need of chewing tobacco. I had no money, and couldn't visit a store for some time because of that red-rope thing. As with every rehab that bans chewing tobacco, I figured how to get a can. I chewed the entire 10 months I was at Sally No. 1 – with the punishment hanging over me that if caught I would lose all my time worked and would have to begin again at Day One. It didn't happen, but I had a couple of very close calls.

The first time, during a period when I kept the can under my wallet in my jeans, one day while exiting the warehouse for a break the tall dorky light-black assistant warehouse supervisor (I usually call him Sleestack) ambushed us with a spot body search. I was second or third in line, almost certainly screwed since we had to "rabbit ear" our pockets – empty them and pull them all the way inside-out for inspection. However the supervisor had to wait for everyone to exit the warehouse before beginning inspections. Couldn't just start the process if a single bennie remained inside hiding a pilfered item. Not one more seemed the gospel. So during this slow-motion filing out, a guy tossed something into a nearby auction cart. The supervisor saw it, and focused his attention on who he suspected was the culprit. That was all the time I needed. I reached into my front pocket and in one smooth move pulled the can out and slipped it into a back pocket, where I gambled that Sleestack wouldn't peek because I was a trusted old white guy. I walked up, pulled up my pants to show my socks, then rabbit-eared my front pockets and looked at him with arms out indicating, "See?" In the past, he had us spin around so he could see our ass pockets, but not this time. He thumbed me down the ramp into the break area, where I had to sit and breathe to slow my thumping heart.

Many months later, I was allowed a rare sick day due to painful gout in an ankle, but decided for whatever reason to go outside to join the fellas during their afternoon break, for coffee and snacks. Walking down, I had the chew again under my wallet, since I never left it behind in the room due to searches. (I literally slept with the can in my underwear briefs at night). As I walked past a ramp at the small chapel where we congregated each morning, the main warehouse supervisor and the house manager, two high-up muck-ety-mucks, were standing at a railing chatting. As I passed, the bald grouchy warehouse manager blurted out, *"What's that in your pocket?!"* At which I patted my wallet bulge and said, "Wallet," and before he could call me over for a closer look, the house manager nudged his elbow and said something that must have been like, *It's okay, he can be trusted.* Like Obi-Wan Kenobi to suspicious stormtroopers in the original *Star Wars*. Haha. I walked outside, a little faster than usual, and shook my head. God, the place was wearing on me.

* * *

After the 44 hours of work each week, around noon each Saturday if you weren't chosen for further punishment in a store, you might still get drafted to work a drop-off collection center on the side of the store. That job equally sucked, mainly due to heat and no shade, and the lifting and carrying of heavy donated items and boxes, but it was better than the stores. I worked our Long Beach store first, which involved mostly keeping clothes off the floor and on racks, and helping move big furniture items that were sold. The first shift was okay, and I'd end up meeting a fellow bennie who became a recurring character over several years. I couldn't even make up a character like that guy, no matter how hard my creative mind works. More on that later. The next week, I was ordered to work at the Torrance store, and my serious displeasure with the Salvation Army began in earnest.

We had just worked many hours of grueling warehouse duties, including four that Saturday morning. Then, we got shipped to a store where the manager and, especially, the assistant manager, were weasels worthy of feature in a *Dilbert* comic strip series. They had no respect whatsoever for us dudes with REHAB stenciled on the back of yellow vests. We were treated like sub-humans. When they tried keeping us working past the 3:30 p.m. end time, because our ride had not yet arrived, I snapped at the assistant manager. "I've already worked eight hours today!" I barked, with a classic *I Mean Business* stare. She insisted, so I spent a few minutes half-hazardly tossing Bric-a-Brac crap onto shelves, with no organization attempted. Just willy-nilly tossing shit everywhere. She asked me to re-shelve returned or misplaced items, which I did, very poorly. After a short period of this song-and-dance, she relieved me.

On all my store shifts, there were always too many of us anyway. I learned to just avoid the managers, whose main job seemed to be punishing us with carrying out huge heavy couches or refrigerators and shit, or just moving stuff around. Like re-organizing an entire row of women's clothes. Make-work shit. We would clear out an entire rack of hanging clothes, and toss it all into yet another big red rolling bin, destined for China. They sat unsold too long, and we had a lot more shit coming in. The waste was extraordinary. I don't know how landfills still have space considering there are three ARCs in the region. The amount of refuse was beyond description. Yet, if you pocketed even a plastic toy ring, you were out of there. Pilfering, they call it.

As I said, one of the first people I met at our store ended up being a re-acquaintance over the following few years. Let's call him Cory. He was funny in the store. He had a tendency to sing out the chorus of the punk anthem "Fuck Authority" by Pennywise randomly. He would even say the "fuck authority" part loud enough for superiors to hear. I never saw him called out for it.

Another was a Navy veteran missing his top four front teeth, which with his thinning tight-cropped hair made him look like a meth addict. He was more like myself, in reality a heavy drinker, who dabbled sporadically in meth. He, too, would resurface many times after our Sally stay. I ended up doing quite a bit of partying all over the place with Cory, and sometimes the Navy vet. He became a truck driver and managed to keep jobs despite sipping beer now and then and teasing his addiction. For a while he drove semis all over the nation, but lost the gig when caught looking at his mobile phone by an in-cab camera (so he says). He dropped down to local routes only, and stayed long at a housing complex for veterans on the west edge of town. He's probably still living there.

As noted, bennies periodically would work a Saturday afternoon at the donation drop-off spot next to the Long Beach store. There, locals would drive up and leave donated items. The gig totally sucked. Way down the road, maybe it was in my second ARC stay, I snuck a couple of airplane bottle shots of vodka with me and drank them during the hours we baked outside waiting to move shit into a trailer. Eventually it took effort to maintain your sanity.

We never seemed to get a decent chunk of down time, though I did find plenty of time to read books. Not long into my stay, I decided on a sponsor from what in AA they called a "group" – a team of dudes and a few chicks who gave themselves the name No Nonsense Group. It would be a choice that had its moments, and provided a ton of AA training, but ultimately created animosity toward the program – a displeasure with AA that remains. Note to AA Nazis: Overdo it, and you might do the opposite of what the program wants most, which is *to collect and keep newcomers*.

It was with that sponsor that I got furthest in the steps, to the beginning of Step 11, attained after a full year of sobriety. Eleven the step is a big book chapter of only a few paragraphs about prayer and meditation. Even though advancing close to that golden final step, I couldn't find the fortitude to even complete the shortest step in the book. Because next was the last step, which essentially means spending the rest of your life finding newcomers to walk through those same 11 steps. By the time I got there, it just wasn't appealing. Somewhere during Step 10, I lost faith in the program and had little confidence that I could instruct newbies about the books and steps, and especially, answering the *how* question. They might ask, *How exactly does it work?* To which I'd probably shrug my shoulders and say something like, "Magic?" Or "Voodoo?" Or … What?

No Nonsense was known by most beneficiaries as a cult. They were strict with sponsorship and constantly had you call, despite the challenges of no mobile phones, and finding quarters and open pay phones. My sponsor was recommended by an older gent who happened to be a colleague of mine from TTC No. 1. Which was such a surprise, since the facilities were located far apart. The dude was my roommate in detox in TTC No. 1. He left after that and did not try residential treatment, thinking he got enough sober time in detox. Like many others learn, he was wrong. Detox just separates you from the chemicals for a short period. Nonetheless, he was a cool older dude and I basically replaced him as a sponsee with the sponsor he'd half-assedly worked with for half a year. The colleague, let's call him Larry, wasn't with me long both times. I appreciated getting help to land a sponsor, since it was required and unlike most everyone else, I took it seriously.

Like other No Nonsense leaders, my sponsor carried multiple sponsees. Being part of the group had some benefits. They often cooked killer meals at a big house in Carson shared by several of them, usually after Sunday "home group" meetings at a closed hospital in Torrance (in which I'd do a brief psyche ward stint, in late 2023, a surreal full-circle moment). There were never many females, but sometimes they'd show up and be very cool, some even attractive.

(I'd learn later, No Nonsense women were strictly off limits, haha). The sponsors seemed to compete to see who could carry the most sponsees, and they were very consistent with fielding phone calls and setting up brief meetings to do "step work," which usually involves reading out loud from AA books (the big book and a smaller "12 Steps and 12 Traditions"). The 12-and-12 was published about 15 years after the big book started AA, and allowed authors the benefit of real experiences to provide more insight into the program, and to offer suggestions in a more understandable manner. Many AA members prefer it to the big book which can seem old and wordy, writing-wise. It is in 12-and-12 where the sponsor concept is introduced; the word is mentioned only once in the big book, in a single story near the end of the book, not really part of The Program and steps. Sponsorship is not a formal part of the AA program. Nowhere in the big book, which contains the actual AA Program, will it say "You must get a sponsor." Sponsors could do pretty much whatever they wanted, and I found the inconsistencies and lack of written instructions unsettling. Some sponsors can actually hurt a newcomer's chances; they need a Hippocratic Oath to do no harm, like doctors.

Being a member of No Nonsense was a drag. You went to more AA meetings with them, often more than required, like up to six a week. Plus, you lost time to car rides back and forth to outside meetings. Often, the Sally hosted AA meetings right inside the facility, an easy way to get signatures on your weekly card. Not for us NN members, though. We had to abide by a weekly schedule of meetings, in San Pedro, Torrance, sometimes other locales, even down in Orange County or way inland. Yet, I stuck with it. Once my brain cleared, I knew I needed serious help and pledged to really try. I had a solid sponsor who would last with me well-past a full year sober, long after I graduated the Sally in September 2015. He kept sponsoring me when I remained living in the Sally for what they would call Phase 2, when graduates remain living there while looking for employment. You still still had to work the warehouse (of course!) but got a day off each week for job searching. Finally I graduated to Phase 3 and wound up in a Sally-linked sober living house in west-center Long Beach near the airport, with a fellow ARC graduate.

A lot of time was wasted at the Sally. Think about how many months. Not only that, it didn't take long to be proved unsafe. A lot of county jail and state prisoners get ordered to complete sentences there. Some rehabs and sober living houses thrived as jails in the region became overcrowded. The government had to reduce jail populations, and pronto. They worked with places like the Sally to take long-time prisoners nearing the end of terms.

About one month into my Sally experience, a beneficiary stabbed another during a dispute in our Bric-a-Brac department. Who knows what the argument regarded, but when a tall, light-skinned and mouthy black kid held up his hands to indicate, "I don't want to fight," my former roommate (and then my current direct co-worker at the sorting table), stabbed him. With one of many knives that landed on the sorting table, my work partner jabbed the victim in the side of the left ribcage, just below the armpit.

Most of the rest of us were in the bathroom washing hands for break, and failed to witness anything. When we exited, I heard someone yell, "He stabbed him!" from somewhere deep in the cavernous building. Then there was a lot of commotion in the other corner of that upstairs work area, near the clothes hanging. I saw a staff member rush the victim to an elevator en route to the lobby and paramedics.

The knife went deep and missed the heart, we learned later, by a quarter-inch. The victim's lung would collapse, and we wouldn't see him again for some time. But we *would* see him, since he was court-ordered. Upon returning he needed a plastic breathing-assist gizmo the rest of the way. He was noticeably more religious.

Something to note here is, the victim was given leeway by the Salvation Army. An alarming thing about the program is, if you get hurt and can't work, you're out. *Even if you get injured due to the work.* You might get a day, maybe two, off for cuts and bruises. But get hurt with an injury that lingers, and out you go. Except when the operation may be liable for the stabbing of a person on their property, of course. That got an exception.

At first, no suspect was identified. The person who eventually would end up the perpetrator actually bitched to staff while they held us upstairs, because *his lunch was being delayed.* They single-filed us down the stairs, down the concrete ramp where I was almost caught with chew, and into the morning chapel room. I walked through the door, past an assistant house manager, who then said the suspect's name aloud and led him away. The suspect had been right in front of me – the big tattooed kid of my first room. He since had been promoted to a two-bed room. Let's call him Adam. He was led to the lobby, where he promptly ran out the front door. He would be captured shortly after at his girlfriend's house. The guy was just finishing a two-year sentence for beating a guy over $120 (for heroin). It seems corrections authorities or the Salvation Army should be careful with violent offenders. Yet there he was, in the middle of a busy sorting operation, none of us wise to his background or temperament. Handling knives and other sharp objects.

Our little crew was locked into the main chapel and each of us was interviewed by police. I thought none of us witnessed it (I would learn years later that one colleague saw it, but feared snitching). I didn't see the act and said so, but added something about work pressure contributing to tension, which got me a subpoena later from the city prosecutor.

After the police interviews, we had an all-beneficiaries meeting in the main chapel, where all the uppity-ups including the warehouse manager were on stage to explain things. When they finished their carefully crafted spiel and asked for questions, I stood and said, "I can't say this *caused* the incident, but I can say that it was *precipitated by work demands*," and sat down. It was true. We were all bludgeoned verbally just before the stabbing by Sleestack, to work harder and faster. Our entire work area was a mess, and he had stopped by to yell at us so much, we were frazzled and working too fast. We didn't dare waste time sweeping; we were whipped into filling as many blue boxes as fast as humanly possible. By the time of the stabbing, we were all totally spent physically and mentally, and dreaded the final shift.

The warehouse manager then jumped forward on stage. He and another Sally official proceeded to scold me. The warehouse man, bald and bespeckled and not very respected, exploded, saying something like, "You're expected to work here. If you don't like it you can leave!" None of his colleagues on stage did or said anything. So there you have how a supposedly Christian organization reacts to honest criticism. The gathering was just for show.

Months later, an administrator who'd moved to the Pasadena ARC visited, and said to me candidly, "*I couldn't believe how they treated you.*" Months later, I got a pass to miss a couple of hours of warehouse work (approval is not automatic) to visit court for my subpoena. Upon arriving, they informed me there was nothing to testify about; the subject pleaded out. The prosecutor considered attempted murder, and the suspect took a deal for seven years in prison, for assault. That was summer 2015 which means the guy should be out of prison. His victim is from a town not far away, who had fingered his attacker while on a stretcher in the lobby because he was mad his kids almost lost their father. As a snitch on a convict, he may not be living comfortably today.

* * *

A subpoena, felony criminal court, snitches and repercussions were not something one dealt with often in Simi Valley. The bad-asses there get arrested, or the cops shoo them away and out of town, usually over the hill to the San Fernando Valley. So just a month in at the Sally, I knew I was no longer in Kansas, so to speak. I also still had five months to go, barring a miracle. As if anyone would drive to Long Beach and rescue me. I was far from friends, but I do admit, the thought of a rescue crossed my mind. I could only imagine the thoughts of prison inmates awaiting some miracle. But at least they didn't have to work full time in a dust-choked warehouse while being yelled at constantly.

I did get to explore a totally new town and environment. I discovered I liked living in a real city, mainly downtown Long Beach a few blocks from the Sally down Alamitos Avenue toward the ocean. With a population of about a half-million, it is considered a big city by federal standards. For comparison, consider the populations of these cities big enough for National Football League franchises. Green Bay, Wisconsin, home of the Packers, has a population of about 250,000, in a market of 471,000 people. Its entire market could fit into Long Beach. The Bills club in Buffalo, N.Y. has a market of some 632,000, from a population of 278,349; and New Orleans is home to 357,767 people, while the Saints' market is 687,000 people. Tack on suburbs connected to Long Beach like Signal Hill, Lakewood, and Bellflower, and Long Beach is big enough to host an NFL team. (Maybe not now, with two franchises calling Inglewood home).

I did not miss the sleepy spread-out suburbs. I really liked beaches, plus downtown had a little marina with a small L-shaped mall with a fake wood boardwalk. I enjoyed walking downtown between the tall buildings. The biggest building in Simi Valley then was five floors, but it's since been demolished. The tallest now I believe is four floors. I became an expert on the public transportation system in and around The LBC, as it is known, for Long Beach, California. Right through the middle of town, from First Street off the shoreline leading due north all the way to Los Angeles, was an above-ground light rail line. The Blue Line was a blast for getting north and south fast; and all the city and regional buses criss-crossed town and ran often. I last had a driver's license in 2013. I walked a lot, and still do. As of this writing, I still don't miss having a car, at all. Except when I want to date, haha. Cars are expensive and cause stress.

Some things were memorable during my first ARC stay. While sorting junk, you'd run across all kinds of stuff, including wads of cash, and a lot of little sponge balls we cannot sell but are great for throwing at dudes from other departments passing by. Once in the Bric, we had this dashing and rather well-built younger guy who we liked for loading, but he didn't like it and somehow got transferred to … *books*. That place had a ginormous pile of old books stacked up constantly, and two guys always sorting through it all. It reminded me of *Fahrenheit 451*. I'd think, just toss kerosene and a match on the pile! Books can't be very profitable, take up a lot of space, and are heavy. That's how I began to evaluate donations, by value vs. weight and trouble.

I honestly don't know what book guys did all day while we broke backs sorting tons of crap. The books gig didn't involve constant lifting, and they seemed to be immune from Sleestack badgering. We Bric guys were not terribly fond of books guys. We considered them soft.

I saved the squishy balls at my station by wedging them between parts of the bottom of the conveyor belt. I could hide three to five at a time, and pretty much always had ammo. One day, I noticed the stylish guy who left us for books at the edge of that department, where ours ended. He was behind one of the dreaded six-foot-tall red rolling bins, and all I could see was the top of his head. He was about 60 feet away, and I had a thick metal support beam in the way. I grabbed a ball, leaned over onto one leg to peek around the beam for a clear sight path, and standing diagonally lobbed it nice and high just hoping to surprise him by hitting the cart. But, nooo. I watched the ball clear the cart, over the top, and the dude's head popped up like a Jack-in-the-Box. Obviously something scared the shit out of him. I ducked down, and peeked over the sorting table at my victim, who walked around the cart and stared at us all. But he didn't ask. Probably because he knew we'd all deny it. Still, I was having a really hard time stifling guffaws. It was Spitball Incident redux.

Later on during break I saw the guy, and said I heard someone hit him with a squishy ball (kind of hinting that it was Cory, who worked way closer). "Yeah," he said. "I was standing there reading a book and it hit me in the middle of my chest."

Warehouse work did not always have to be not fun. Those red rolling carts were tall and we stored empty ones side by side waiting to be filled with junk. Much of the time there was this huge farm of them, like gigantic Lego blocks squished together. I learned to push narrow paths between some, zig-zagging a little so no one could see me from the opening, and create little room-like nooks. Then I'd bring an egg crate back there to sit and read. When serving as a runner I spent a lot of time in a nook, basically listening to the crew in case it got busy, or Sleestack visited. That guy was known to sneak around and spy on us, so it was cool returning the favor and secretly eyeing him wherever he was slithering off to. From my sitting position I could see his shiny bald head bouncing by.

In June, I ran across a little pendant that looked real pretty. It had a tiny dove set over a heart, and at that time I was just beginning to emulate everyone around me, which meant pilfering. Guys there would steal so much gold, they would walk down the street and pay to rent a private business post office box to store all the goods since our rooms and lockers were searched consistently. Getting caught with pilfered items was a really big offense. It could mean ejection. Nonetheless I always wore brief-style underwear, and you could hold quite a bit under your balls, if you wrapped packages in plastic bags or such. If I knew a particular day might be heavy on loot, I'd wear two pairs of underwear for support. I got good at walking with things tucked down low.

Sleestack did searches often, usually at the end of the day when we were sweaty and pooped and ready for fresh air. It always was a drag. I saw guys get caught all sorts of ways, from wearing three pairs of tees under their col-lared shirt (we had to wear collared shirts tucked in at all times on property), to having rings in a shoe, or something tucked into a waistband. *Rookies*, I thought. They might pat you down, but *they won't pat under your balls*.

One day a pair of surf shorts plopped onto the table, and attached was a little bag made of thick clear plastic, with a double-zip closing mechanism. It was about the size of a large mobile phone, tethered to the shorts to hold car keys, cash, or small valuables while the surfer was in the water. Well, chewing tobacco cans have metal tops, and one day the house manager after our final shift introduced a hand-held metal detector we called The Wand. Yes, the mega-rich Salvation Army took pilfering extremely seriously. And we took our pilfering seriously. It felt like a Tom and Jerry cartoon, and they were always Tom the cat, getting bamboozled by Jerry the mouse.

I got lucky that day, because either I was out of chew, or just forgot to sneak in a can. Sometimes a can would slip out of the briefs and start sliding down a leg. At which point I would calmly go to the bathroom and put it back where it belonged. That day, because I had no chew can with a metal top, by luck I passed the first Wand test. Some dude with cigarettes got caught due to the foil inner lining of packs; plus he had a lighter which was forbidden in the warehouse. That guy was pissed: two weeks with a yellow lanyard trapped on property.

With the Wand, I had to figure out how to get chew in and out of the warehouse. And I got lucky, with the thick pouch with double Ziplocks. You could fit two full cans of chew into that thing, and squish it flat so it rested easier in your underwear and wouldn't slip out. That thing was awesome, and I had it for months and filled it often. Guys knew and would ask for a dip and I'd hand them my pouch, and they'd run to the bathroom and back. A lot of shenanigans happened in the restrooms, for sure. Remember, if caught with chew, it was automatic start-over. One respected dude had about 90 days under his belt and got caught chewing, and had to start over. He was court-ordered so he had to eat it and ended up doing nine months for a Get Out of Jail certificate.

Back to the little gold heart with the dove. That was the first item I thought to pilfer, which I did for no particular reason, but later decided to mail it to my youngest daughter who had visited earlier with my father. I wrote my letter and dropped the pendant in there, I think even using Scotch tape to secure it a little so it wouldn't slide around in the envelope, and dropped it off at the front desk for them to mail. That was my big error.

The new house manager decided that day to shake outgoing letters.

Surprise! Mine had a little weird weight in it, was opened, and I was busted. They called me in and asked to see a receipt, which we are advised to do when buying items from outside. I argued that I bought it but forgot to ask for a receipt, but that I'd be happy to go back to that store and get one! I even put my offer in writing.

Which probably got me an additional week. They weren't buying it and I wore the yellow rope for three weeks. I learned later that they might be lenient if you just confess. Looking back, I'm lucky I didn't get the full-month yellow rope, which is a very serious offense, like putting you on the verge of ejection. The yellow rope was like a Scarlet Letter, only it was the Golden Letter, or maybe Lemon Letter.

I don't remember getting into any other trouble there, both stints, except the ending of stay No. 2. In the first, I made it to September and graduated – not before a bowling ball rolled off the sorting table and landed right next to my foot, actually touching my shoe but not crushing bones. That would have gotten me kicked out a week before graduating, by this Christian church. I agreed to do Phase 2 and keep working for the room and meals while job hunting. I did this all of September and October, into November. I was at one of their two computer stations all the time, whenever I walked by and noticed one unused. We also used computers at the library two blocks away. For the longest time I just couldn't find a job, or at least one I could work under the Sally's rules. Getting a job meant Phase 3, working while you lived there, but skipping the warehouse or truck work. That started in November before Thanksgiving.

One night arriving back from a No Nonsense group meeting, I saw an open PC and decided to use the last minutes before the 10 p.m. lights-out to search Craigslist. By then I'd gotten my process of sending my resume or LinkedIn profile link rapid-fire to several employers over a brief period, often forgetting which jobs I'd applied for (and why). Apparently I'd responded to a part-time job ad for the Queen Mary, an old British cruise ship permanently docked at the end of the Los Angeles River. It was a tourist attraction, for reasons I don't understand. To me it's just an old rust bucket. The newer cruise ships dock next to it and absolutely dwarf the Queen Mary – double in size. And the Queen Mary never un-docked.

They bit and emailed the next day, and said they were hosting a "job fair" on the ship the following day, a Sunday. Luckily it was in the afternoon because no way any of us got out of chapel Sunday mornings. I returned from church, stripped off my monkey suit, put on jeans and a collared shirt and walked and bused way out to the Queen Mary. I was pleasantly surprised, the bus ride was not bad. It wasn't really a job fair, just tables inside an open area right when you entered from a wide ramp from the shore. Who knows what that open area was in the cruising heyday. The Queen Mary was big enough to transport troops in World War II. There were three or four fold-out tables with people in bright-colored polo shirts sitting behind them. I approached the one with no line, where a tall, skinny black guy sat. He was super friendly, asked a few questions, and it started to feel kind of like an interview. He had me fill out an application as we spoke, and as soon as I was done, he thanked me and said they'd call. It lasted maybe 15 minutes.

He explained the job was as an usher at a seasonal special event they staged called "Chill," with rides and attractions, the biggest of which was a huge ice box where a Chinese team sculpted slides and human-sized figures to depict the entire story of Charles Dickens' "A Christmas Carol" – a scene at a time, room after room, all in ice. The Ice Kingdom was gnarly to see, let alone work in. Anyway, a day later they called (probably via a phone I'd snuck in by then) and said I was hired. I started when it opened, the Friday before the weekend preceding Thanksgiving. I'd end up working about 20 hours a week, mostly night shifts like 5 to 10 p.m., which I loved because it got me out of the Sally building a lot – and out of many No Nonsense meetings.

They gave us a single polo shirt, for people expected to work four or five shifts a week. Never understood that, but since I lived among slobs, I didn't mind using the shirt all week. It was covered by my black jacket, or the coat they provided to work inside the Ice Kingdom. It was cold outside, but nothing compared with the 6 degrees inside the Kingdom. When they assigned shifts they'd indicate in advance what role you'd be assigned, so you'd know how many Kingdom shifts you had to survive. Some shifts would just be ushering outdoors, like through mazes, or pushing the world's largest rocking horse up and down while people sat atop it (I'm not making this up). Ushering I found easy, and the freedom to walk around the ice rink, or past exhibits, was fun. It was almost always crowded, and provided a Christmas feel I hadn't experienced in years. I worked with much younger adults, mostly college students with theater aspirations, and their enthusiasm energized me. I'm still friends on Facebook with some. I kept thinking, this is the best job I've ever had. I enjoyed working there. A lot.

Phase 3 allowed me to work as much as I wanted, and I got special permission to return after 10 p.m. if work demanded. Which was weird, because the old Sally building was eerily quiet after lights-out and they breathalyzed me walking in even though I was coming straight from work and straight to bed. I could stay living there for three paychecks, or for two months. That gave me a target to plan my escape. I could save money and get into a sober living house, which I'd done before, albeit briefly.

Plus I wanted to see my mother over Christmas, and to do so, I'd have to not be in the Sally, which didn't allow overnight passes. I had a month to figure it out. My mother had been diagnosed with pancreatic cancer in October, which Dad informed me of when I called for her birthday Nov. 12. She had months to live, he said. Just absolutely shocking news to hear over your little free welfare phone standing in the dark in front of an elementary school in a strange new town. Considering the months of Sally beatdowns I endured, I thought to myself, *"How much more can I possibly take?"*

Thank goodness I was locked up with random UAs. Home was too far away to attempt Simi Valley and back by 10. I pressed ahead with work. I wanted out of the Sally before Christmas. My sponsor closely monitored my progress, and I still attended a lot of AA meetings with him, even though I missed a few due to work (haha). I'd have daytime downtime without working the warehouse, so sometimes I used a PC there to pretend to be looking for work while I checked emails and set fantasy baseball team lineups. Somewhere along the line I found and applied for a job at the headquarters of a chain of custom closet franchises that needed a social media manager. I applied for that position, but they saw my LinkedIn profile and said they had a bigger role in mind for me: marketing manager specifically for home builders. It was a full-time job, I interview well, and was hired. It didn't start until mid-December, and I decided to keep working nights at Chill, until it ended 10 days into January. For a few weeks I'd have no days off, and sometimes worked 12 or more hours in a day. And I loved it.

* * *

I spent so much time at the Salvation Army, I could go on and on about memories. I had to think hard to memorialize only those important to share. All ARCs have these officers who wear white uniforms, acting like it was real military. Always a high-ranking officer would be in charge of the overall operation. A business manager might be in charge of generating income any way possible, but some adult in a Navy-like white uniform was the property's top dog. That first stay, it was a major, an old Filipino dude who served along with his wife who also had to wear the white uniform, long skirt version. The guy was an unpopular jackass. Each new guy was called in for a sit-down, where he talked about Jesus and Christianity. I remember telling him I grew up Catholic, with a grandmother who taught at a private Catholic school for 26 years, and he said Catholicism is not Christian. He said Catholics worship Mary, not Jesus. So he quickly lost me, though I admit learning more about the Bible than ever before. That wasn't such a bad thing. The overarching theme for the Bible is *love*; the books are full of instructions and teachings to help people live better. How could anyone oppose that? To this day, I apply lessons learned from chapel services, the Bible, and AA meetings. I'm not the same person as I was before this whole recovery odyssey.

Once again most memorable were the characters. I mentioned Cory and the Navy vet-truck driver. There was a little guy from Texas who thought he looked like Superman, who ended up working beside me for months sorting junk. He thought we were friends, but in reality I found him annoying especially near the end. He just talked nonstop, about meaningless shit. And I was stuck at my station forced to listen.

Other characters included a bad young heroin addict who constantly talked about doing hard drugs and overdosing; and another young guy about his age who played bass in the chapel band. For a spell, they both moved shit around in our department. They got into a shoving match once, but neither was disciplined.

There was this buff con who'd been there before, who acted like no one could take him on, and he might or might not have been correct. There was this groovy kid from San Luis Obispo who played guitar well and sang leading the chapel band. Eventually Cory got in trouble for finding and wearing the ugliest sports coat imaginable in chapel, and the major called him out for it – a humorous exchange where Cory had to stand and look down at his coat. Within days, Cory had a new coat, but the groovy band leader was wearing that ugly grey plaid sucker in front of everyone in the chapel. He did it every week, and it was hilarious. There was a guy about my age named Mark, who would join me in both Sally visits, sharing the same sponsor for my second tour. He's the one who would be discovered dead outdoors in Torrance not long thereafter. He was a terrible alcoholic. There was a heavyset gay cook-in-training who worked the kitchen who everyone liked, and I was pretty solid friends with him for a long time. I see him on Instagram now and then; he's lost so much weight he's almost unrecognizable. He looks happy and I'm way stoked for him. He was the person who loaned me $20 to eat one time in 2017, money mentioned in the chapter on that horrible year for me.

* * *

I secured a sober living house bed through a Sally contact, and walked out on Dec. 22, a few days shy of 10 months in custody. Looking back, it seems insane considering how much I endured. So much time. There just was not much of a recovery focus there, aside from my personal efforts with my sponsor. The warehouse work was back-breaking, demeaning, and supervised by seriously mean, borderline sadistic weasels. I packed up and got my clothes into the sober living house, stayed a day or so, then took off for Simi Valley to see Mom. Mom looked okay, and was in decent spirits, happy to see me finally, but it was clear she was ill. It all was very difficult to digest, after all I survived all year, to have God make my mother suffer. I stayed at their place every other weekend until she finally passed, on March 1, 2016.

All the while I was commuting a decent distance every day by bus, train, then another bus, into an area of south Los Angeles called Athens. There, in what is known as the Willowbrook area, about 9,000 people lived. It didn't feel unsafe, but the memory is of dreary old suburb houses and warehoused businesses and a load of car traffic. The custom closet company job at first was interesting, since I would create an entirely new endeavor. I had freedom to be creative, and arranged from scratch a decent marketing outreach program for owners and managers of franchises nationwide to plug-and-play to reach new home builders. At an all-franchises conference in late January, I offered a Power Point presentation that was received well. The new owners of the Oregon franchise approached and said it was exactly what they were looking for. The company sold new closet projects to homeowners directly, but sometimes got bulk orders from land developers constructing new houses. My job was to help reach these developers, hopefully prior to construction of new-home projects. If it worked, a franchise might get an order for numerous closets in one location – multiple closets, great profit potential. I prepared a complete guidebook and emailed it to them all, and we were just starting to get on our way.

* * *

When Dad called to report Mom's passing, I was on a subway rail platform, waiting to train home. I took the news, hung up, and stood there just numb. I didn't move for some time, then somewhere on the spot decided I wouldn't change anything in my routine. I would keep plugging away with work and AA, because that's what Mom would have wanted. I was sober the last time I saw her, and it inspired me to keep it up. I took a one-year sobriety cake before she passed, and my sponsor forced me to speak before a big crowd in a new meeting where we knew no one. No Nonsense, pffft. I was deep into the steps, working on Steps 9 and 10, calling my sponsor every morning per his orders, before even getting on the first bus. It began to get tiresome, and as we approached Step 12, I started having suspicions about a future with AA. I lasted about a month after Mom's death. As with almost all relapses, I don't know what happened. It began innocently enough with a beer, maybe two. I think it happened on a date – and yes, I shouldn't have been dating.

The 9th Step is where you try to make amends. For the step prior, you write a list of all people you'd harmed *in your life*, and you had to be "willing to make amends to them all." Then, in Step 9, you started making those amends, usually by phone. My 8th step always seems to end up with about 65 people, things, or institutions (like the IRS, which I wondered about but never got around to). My sponsor had me start that process, but instead of staying stuck in Step 9 while I made all the amends, we moved on into the next step, to do them simultaneously. I never finished that 9th, but I did make some calls. To this day I regret not calling my mother first, since I never got around to doing it. I called my old friend Doug to apologize for just not being a good friend, and he said he didn't feel harmed, we were good. Then, he said in a classic Doug way, "Wait a minute. So you're saying *you have to do anything I ask?*" I guess so, I said. "Then you have to go to a David Gilmour concert with me." I guess so, I tentatively agreed. Haha. I went on Easter, and enjoyed the show, though as a punk rocker now it can be hard to get into '70s-like slow tunes. My friend Brad was with Doug, visiting from Vegas to see the Pink Floyd legend again. I waved down to Doug and Brad and their wives when we saw each other, but I never did get to go talk with Brad. It would be the last time I saw him, before he passed a few years later from Lou Gehrig's disease. He'd moved to Texas, and by then I was so deep into my shit I never did figure out a way to visit.

At the concert, I did manage to meet up with Doug and his wife Cheri for a brief visit post-show outside the Forum in Inglewood. Doug said he was sorry to hear about my mother, and I thanked him and said I was just trying to keep doing what I was doing, stay in a routine. I was with a date at the time who never seemed to get over how I didn't seem to mourn Mom's death enough, and she mentioned that to my friends. That was the last time I saw her.

The problem was, the routine then wasn't entirely healthy. I had dropped my sponsor and diligent AA work, and was on my own. What a major fuck up. I'd find spots of temporary relief from what was growing into a lot of anxiety, especially about work demands, Mom's death, and the then-light drinking. A girlfriend named Robin helped much, to relieve stress with her humor and silliness. Today, I probably could identify such a perfect storm of troubles, but during that period I was clueless. I thought I was fine, and I was not, simple as that. I really needed to be engaged with a professional to get past the initial grief. But I chose to brave it alone.

My drinking increased daily, as usual, and I was ejected from the sober living home – shortly after my roommate assaulted me one night while in bed. I vaguely remember walking into our darkened room, where he was having sex with someone, and I said something before curling up in my bed facing away. I vaguely remember his angry face, before blacking out. He punched down to hit me, four times in the face, and I had a big black eye during the whole transition out of there. That included during my very first stay at a psyche ward, in Bellflower, and an initial meeting with the manager of a new sober living house in north Long Beach. That sober living stay was brutally bad, but I would learn two years later that it was not even close to the worst sober living house. That easily was Sherry's House in Compton.

Immediately upon leaving the first Long Beach sober living house, I barely remember spending a few days hanging out in a hotel room with Robin, drinking and more. Eventually she decided to go home, and I didn't hear from her again until 2019. I'm so happy we've reconnected; she lives in Reno with plans to visit me in Hawaii one day.

Dad came to the rescue and drove to Bellflower to save me from the psyche ward, where I was given a list of sober living houses in the area. While in his truck, I connected with the manager of one with a bed open. (I'd quickly learn why). Dad agreed to fund the first month, and just like that I was living on Market Street in north LBC not far off Atlantic Avenue. That house manager for some reason thought Dad was loaded and could be counted on for rent in case I turned out to be a fuck up. (Which of course I was).

A month in, it was clear I couldn't make rent. I'd been spending wildly, dining at fine nearby eateries, and gulping gallons of booze. The apartment, neighborhood, and whole operation was too terrible to take. One morning I fell hard running across Market and smashed my head on a curb, bleeding so profusely the house manager said he'd seen gunshot victims bleed less. It cost me two days in a hospital in a neck brace, with a really nasty upper-left forehead scar that took years to fade. Eventually time ran out, and I walked out of the old converted motel, and down the hill to the Sally. A real walk of shame.

* * *

Salvation Army No. 2 began with a seizure the second day. To pass intake, you had to be clean and sober for five days. I already knew the rule, so when asked I said five days clean and sober. Luckily I passed the intake breath test for alcohol. They immediately stuck me right back into the same slot sorting junk at the Bric table, and on the second day during the final break, I sat on a plastic chair outside and seized up. What a horrible, terrifying experience.

In all, the ARC re-do was about 150 days, before ejection for failing a pee test after warehouse work. During this stay, I did not take anything seriously, especially AA. I did the bare minimum number of AA meetings, all in-house, if I did them at all. I forged signatures of phantom AA meeting secretaries on the little paper slip, which we had to submit each Friday to get our weekly cash pay of $3 to $12. I found the most mellow surf-dude sponsor who would visit once a week and shoot the shit and sign my card. I dabbled in pilfering like everyone else. I sipped vodka from airplane bottles many nights. In short, I prepped myself for an inevitable disaster.

Being in a rehab and really not wanting to be there is brutal – especially if you end up in a rehab you already attended. There is a difference between not believing you have a substance abuse problem, and just not desiring to spend all the time in residential treatment. By June 2016, I already had five rehab experiences, so my confidence in their ability to make me better was low. My attitude was, I *expected them* to fix me. I didn't take into account the focus and energy I would have to contribute. For this Sally stay, I felt burned out from a series of things that would have traumatized most any human being. I felt I had PTSD, though physicians always rejected this opinion. The rehabs, hundreds of strangers around me at all times, the violence and threats, the homelessness, the psyche ward, crappy sober living houses, emergency rooms, and more. No excuses though. Once the brain fog cleared and I accepted my fate sorting junk every day, my attitude was set. I would just *do time*. Using my new knowledge of this whole system, I would do the least amount possible, and cruise through half a year while trying to figure out a better way to live life.

For five months I did that. I went through the usual four-bed room, and stayed a decent amount of time in a three-bed room with guys who remain friends on social media to this day. I don't remember drinking while with them because of the odor and tight quarters. I remember doing well with those guys and trudging through days and weeks of work and chapel. That place has much in common with the movie "Ground Hog Day." Seriously repetitive with the work and meal regiment every day, the chapel services, all the guys dressed silly, sillier haircuts, the rules. Oh, so many rules. Like, no facial hair except mustaches. No shaved heads, but only peach fuzz lids allowed. Let your hair grow to near a half-inch and you might get in trouble. I looked like a cop pretty much the whole time, not good walking among weirdos of Long Beach.

The turning point was when they transferred me to a big seven-bed room, a space formerly occupied only by incoming beneficiaries. It was supposed to be temporary, while awaiting improvements to my former hallway of rooms. They planned to make those rooms rentable for good former clients. I heard later that didn't last long.

The seven-bed room sucked. The good news was my old buddy Joe of Brooklyn from my first stay was in there. He too seemed burned out from the previous experience and ready to cruise. And not long after, ol' Cody the recurring character turned up. I didn't notice a quiet young kid in the corner who worked in the kitchen, and that word from him to his co-worker would get to the kitchen manager which would get us pee-tested. Cody ensured my demise by drinking airplane shots openly in the room at night, right across from the snitch kitchen worker.

When Cody arrived he was red-roped on restriction. Passing him in the upstairs recreation-gathering room his first day, I asked if he wanted some booze. I had been sporadically sneaking the airplane bottles inside by tucking them into my socks when checking back into the facility. I was an old white guy who didn't raise suspicions and I took advantage. When you returned from being out, you blew into a tube to prove sobriety, then ran upstairs to your room. Very rarely did they search or Wand you. Bennies worked the front desk mostly, and they either were too busy, or lazy. Once I provided Cody with a couple of little bottles, all the sudden I was sneaking in multiple shots every day, like three in each sock every afternoon. I would drink in the hallway bathroom and return to my bed to read, very careful with the empty bottles to take with me in the morning to secretly dump in the trash outside. Sometimes staff searched trash cans, we knew. We were always under suspicion.

I lived in that big room for about a week. The vodka intake at night increased little by little, but I read a lot and managed. My bed was close to the front door, and one time the assistant house manager walked in, looked left, then right (in my direction), and inhaled hard a few times, making sure we knew he was sniffing to smell. As if to message, *We know something's up.* I should've taken the hint. I also was unaware that they now could detect alcohol in your urine for 48 to 72 hours. Apparently at least traces stay in your bladder. News to me, and I'd passed urine samples for years by then.

Finally one day sorting at the Bric table, two airplane bottle shots of tequila rolled out of a box. I grabbed them quickly, hid one under the table, and then walked the other over to Cody, who was at the end of the conveyor belt grabbing priced items to box for shipment to stores. They called break, and I hit the bathroom and slugged a shot, expecting Cody would do the same. I walked to the break area and drank some coffee to top it off, and had a groovy last shift. I'd already completed all the notebook work required each month, and had a post-work meeting with my counselor scheduled. I was nearing the end of this drudgery, and looked forward to getting signed off for completing five months.

After work we marched down that ramp and into that same small chapel room, and the staff was there which was noteworthy. Usually we high-tailed it straight upstairs to change and check out. The house manager said he was announcing UAs for the day. My name was on the list. I shrugged and went upstairs, like no big deal. I grabbed my now-thick binder carrying months of program work, and headed downstairs to pee before my counselor meetup. When they announced the UAs, they said we could do it immediately, or after dinner which would have at least bought hours of time. I was cocky and said I'd be there in a few minutes.

Of course I failed the UA, and immediately contested it. I just worked eight hours, how possibly could I have drank alcohol up in the warehouse all day? I demanded a lab test, as the plastic cups have a reputation for false positives. Standard operating procedure for Rehab All-Stars. I sat in a windowed conference room awaiting my fate, while client colleagues walked by wide-eyed knowing it was a big deal. The overall program director told the house manager they would send the UA to a lab for testing, but if I still failed, I could not return to the Salvation Army ever. Fine, I said.

Just about to turn to return to my room, the house manager said, "Oh yeah, one more thing. Give me your badge." My green rope. I'd have to wear yellow, in restriction, until the results returned. Fuck that, I gave him my green rope, indicated I was leaving, and high-tailed it upstairs to get my shit. They quickly followed, because the rule was if you graduated you could keep the clothes they provided, but those ejected could not. It was right before Thanksgiving and cold outside, but they refused to let me take the jacket. Not even my own underwear. It was what I was wearing only. Somehow I talked them into letting me take a long-sleeved purple flannel shirt. That mercy would prove valuable.

By this time the drinking bug was well on its usual way, making me more thirsty each day. I couldn't wait to get out the front door and down to a store for vodka. Sure, I was shocked at what just transpired, but fuck it, I was thirsty and wasn't all that interested in staying. I stopped at their adjacent store and bought a backpack, and for some reason left my phone in the backpack. (A reason I raced to my room after handing over my green rope was to get to the bathroom up there to get my phone hidden high up atop a fluorescent light box). Then I proceeded to drink hard down Alamitos Avenue, bouncing along, when my inebriated brain decided drugs would be fun. I met some street dude who said he could get some, and I followed him around for quite some time zig-zagging down alleys and even through a building's upstairs hallway. Finally I said I had to pee, so I set my bag down and walked a few feet around a corner to do it. Of course when I returned he was gone. Gone was my phone, plus jewelry loot from the warehouse. At that point it was just me, my jeans, a thin shirt, the purple flannel, and a little cash. Unsure if I had a ball cap or not. It was very chilly even in the early evening.

I have no idea what I did that night. I woke up the next morning on the porch of an apartment building all the way down Alamitos south, then east a little on Broadway. It was a small landing porch elevated up some five steps, and someone opening the front door woke me. She gave me a weird look as if saddened. I looked down to see my purple flannel and dorky white sneakers, then up to see sunlight. Shit, I thought. I wobbled to my feet and trudged westward toward downtown proper.

That was followed by a couple days of very hard drinking, with slight memories of buying a thick camouflage jacket, and sitting not too far up the street from the Sally shitfaced drunk on Thanksgiving afternoon, at a picnic table with a bennie who was commiserating with me. These would be the very first actions in what would end up being the worst 13-month stretch of my life.

A few weeks later, Cody was ejected, a real Rehab All-Star. Before he got in for his second stay, I had called him from the Sally (somehow!) and asked him to go to the Market Street sober living complex and retrieve my laptop and Doc Marten boots. All the rest – a nice clothing collection from 10 months of trading in old for new at the Sally store – he could leave. He agreed and did so.

Months later when I finally came to, I emailed and texted him to retrieve my property. No responses, so I looked up his last name in Gardena, and gambled that a guy with the same last name was related. So I trained and bused there, quite a trek. Sure enough, Cody was there, drunk and asking to walk to a liquor store to buy him a beer. I was sober, only wanting my stuff and a return to the LBC. Cody took me along some railroad tracks to drink, where he told me my items were gone. He sold the laptop and boots. For booze, maybe drugs, no doubt. That laptop had been a gift from a client to use to promote her work and books, a gig I secured while with Shannon in Fillmore. That and the boots, gone. I shrugged and walked back to the train. Why I even maintained contact with Cody is beyond my comprehension.

Back to the end of 2016. After Thanksgiving, a couple of weeks later I came to just enough to pursue something I learned from others on the streets. The county welfare office would provide a week in a hotel if you had food stamps, which I did. I stayed briefly in a clean hotel room funded by the county, in a killer location just a block off Ocean Boulevard. During this time I ran into the same guy who had stolen my backpack the night I exited the Sally, and I proceeded to party with him in a room at the infamous Club Motel on Lime until he stole my stuff again while I slept. I then scuffled on the streets for a bit until walking into an emergency room because I was crazily exhausted. I claimed chest pains. They had to take me, I knew, insurance or not. After several hours they discharged me, at like 1 a.m. the next morning, homeless and into a brutal rain storm. I walked a half block, found a covered hospital delivery area, and plopped down on bare concrete to sleep. It was raining too hard to walk anywhere. The area was well-lit, and the rain made it bitterly cold. I lasted about an hour before walking right back into the ER to fib, claiming I just coughed up blood.

They did the intake as expected, and took vitals, which triggered very surprised reactions. Same nurses. One said, "Did you just leave here and do meth?" I said no, that I felt just like when I left. They said my blood pressure was stroke level, and that I would be *admitted*. For four days they held me, under constant surveillance. At one point, a nurse ran in because my blood pressure dipped dangerously *low*. No one knew the cause. They eventually chalked it up to some nervous system misfiring. At least I did get to call Dad from the hospital bed on Christmas, telling him of my heart issues. He was mad and disinterested.

Soon after, I discovered the city's winter shelter was opening, and that's where the worst year of my life began. I never did rehab in 2017, by stubborn choice. All year, very purposely I fought against returning to a rehab, and it almost killed me. My anger at the Sally and the rehabs and AA was fierce, as if they were to blame for my failures. In this book I try to avoid providing too much of what in recovery they call "war stories" – absurd tales of drinking and using and the debauchery that goes with it. However, I will outline details of how 2017 progressed, because it serves as an example of what can happen when a bad addict fights against revisiting rehabs. Rehabs might be painful, but life can get much, much worse.

SPECIAL REPORT
NO REHAB, 2017

Odyssey of the Absurd

Years later, a World War I film with horrid battle scenes was released, and I raced to see it. I love history, especially anything to do with America's wars. I chuckled when I first saw the movie title, because it was rare for a film to have just a number for the title; but also because with all the blood and carnage, "1917" reminded me of a single year that was more gruesome than any other personally. It happened to be exactly 100 years after that year of the War to End All Wars. The year 2017 was unimaginably horrific.

In summary, that year featured stints hanging out with two prostitutes, one older and (kind of) retired from the business, the other an active call girl around age 50 who wouldn't accept anything less than $100 per session. Both were addicted to heroin, the former injecting it, while the latter smoked it almost nonstop off foil. The semi-retired hooker I learned later was bipolar and would vanish for weeks at a time, only to return in surprising fashion, over and over like a bad dream. She injected me in September 2017 after hours of drinking vodka, and I overdosed – yet survived thanks to her speedy actions.

That was months away from the inauspicious beginning of 2017, when I spent the first two-and-a-half months living in a winter shelter. After many weeks of homeless drudgery, I won an unemployment case and used the money to live in a hotel room with my new shelter friend the semi-retired prostitute; then very briefly (a week) relocated to the Valley via a former editor friend who tried to help; then immediately afterward spent a week in a rented northwest Valley room before being ejected for offering meth to my roommate fresh out of jail and on probation. Sometime around there, I stayed in a Van Nuys hotel, did meth and drank, and was cited one night for solicitation of prostitution. Not knowing what the hell I was doing, I followed an attractive latina back into darkness and an awaiting police sting. It took an odyssey of long train and bus rides to a San Fernando courthouse in Sylmar to address the citation.

The first stay with the semi-retired hooker was where my meth addiction began, in mid-March 2017. I had the unemployment case money and she had connections nearby. We'd wake each morning and she would call in orders of $40 worth of dope – half in black, half in white, for her heroin and my meth. The first time I did heroin was when she injected me the first full day together. The next day she shot me with a goofball, a mix of the two drugs, which was intense, to put it mildly. Then the money started to run out and she sneaked away, I thought forever. Then came weeks of blurry memories, like the appearance of the old editor, the very short stays at two places, the Van Nuys citation, and other misdeeds.

After a brief yet quite rough stay living at a train station in the northwest Valley, I called Dad and he came to the rescue. Upon exiting the train station, I noticed he was driving the opposite direction of Simi Valley. I asked, and he said he was taking me somewhere to put distance between us. That ended up being a Motel 6 on Pacific Coast Highway in Long Beach around the inception point of Hookers Row. He purchased seven days, provided some cash, and said it should be enough to get my shit together and find somewhere to live. I did try a little, but mostly just partied hard. The semi-retired prostitute returned, and stayed a few days until I had a severe psychosis episode one evening and sleep-walked right over her in her bed. I literally walked over her and her bed en route to the door, which I opened to peer out into the darkness to see 118 on the door – and realize the reality of being in a hotel room in the wee hours. I went back to bed.

The next morning I had no recollection, only that I had the worst dream ever and it seemed to last forever. I scared the hell out of her, and she once again left. The week purchased by Dad ended, and out I went to wander. At least I had a better night climate. Except for land close to the ocean, most

LBC temperatures were mild at night. Still, the winter shelter had ended and there was no money or night-time roof.

One day sitting on a shoreline grassy slope leaning against my backpack sipping my last half-pint of vodka, the old editor friend called surprisingly. I told him exactly where I was sitting and what I was looking at (the ocean), and what I was sipping. He said by the end of the week his wife would be gone for some time, so I could get there by Friday and stay a spell and get my shit together. Sound familiar?

I had a few days to kill and he offered to purchase a hotel room, which I found for a decent deal up at the south end of North Long Beach, which in reality is south Compton and not like the rest of The LBC. This room was nice, designed for a wheelchair, with a huge bathroom with big Spanish-like tiles all around and marble around the tub. In other words, way too nice for this troublemaker. Somehow I had some dough – I think the editor wired a little spending money for food and the like – so I scored an enormous sack of meth from a black guy named Bird who I met shortly after the solicitation incident in Van Nuys. It's amusing how you freely trade numbers with street strangers. Think about it: you really don't want your number saved on a dealer's phone. He called, I trained out to the Valley to meet up, and in a rather sketchy drive around in his van he asked to borrow $200 (after I already paid for the ice). I said I didn't have any extra dough, even though it was hidden inside the band of my ball cap. Bird was interesting. He lived way out in the North Los Angeles County desert, well beyond Mohave, and commuted all over the region to sling dope and manage prostitutes. A dedicated businessman.

I remember a while after that exchange, a black gal messaged me cold, and we began conversing before she explained we met during that first meeting with Bird. She had been sitting in the passenger seat of a huge old gas-guzzler sedan Bird parked, where I walked up to ask to score. I had no cash when the girl later messaged, or there is potential I would have met up. I was so mentally out of it. For some reason, once free of career and family obligations, I behave like a rock star and can get into the debauchery I read about for years. It's a strange phenomenon.

Back at the North Long Beach hotel room, I managed to make a couple of clinic appointments, to follow up with treatment for a urinary tract infection probably caused by a hernia, and some other ailment I can't remember. Externally, I might have looked okay, sniffing small amounts of meth in the morning to wake up, but never over-doing it. I knew to clean up at least some before going out in public. However, inside, my body was not doing well. I just kept snorting crushed ice, making appointments, and somehow searching the internet for a place to live. After responding to a few Craigslist ads, I was called by a property owner who interviewed me for a bed at her eastside sober living complex, about two miles east of the Sally down Anaheim Street.

She arranged an in-person visit with the property manager the next afternoon, which meant … no meth or vodka deep into the day. Uh-oh. I think I met her there at like 1:30 p.m., and I was jonesing badly. I tried to clean up, and hoped for no trembling hands, but I must have looked at least a little shaky to this person who lived around addicts. She had never seen me before, to have something to compare against, which probably helped through the half-hour interview and intake process. She said I could move in any time, but I delayed a day, knowing I had another night funded at the hotel. One last night of partying, my brain directed. I still had a big rock of meth, and couldn't bring it into a sober living house. Could I?

The next morning, I checked out of the hotel but had hours to kill before the property manager would be home from work to allow access. I dragged my big bag to the bus and down to Bixby Park on the bluffs overlooking the beach and ocean. Just killing time, after smoking some pot with a random gay dude who sat with me on a little park knoll, and sprinkling some meth on top of his pot in a small container before he slithered away, I jumped on the bus up Cherry to my new home just off PCH. Getting on the bus with a huge pack on my back, I took a big step up and it was the first time

I felt something down near my groin. That hernia would not be fixed until triple-hernia surgery in Hawaii in 2022.

I was a little high, sore, and physically drained when I entered the new sober living complex. I was set live upstairs in a two-bed room down the hall from the daughter (with her husband) of the house manager. The manager lived in an apartment with its own entry adjacent to but not connected with our house. Yet we all shared a living room and kitchen. Overall, it was nice and cozy. My roommate was out of state for a spell, and when he returned he soon was kicked out for weird behavior. I would run into him later. He ended up staying temporarily in a North Long Beach hotel room with … my dealer. Talk about awkwardness. I walk in to score, and there's my former roommate in a very small hotel room with my dealer and his girlfriend.

My new roommate was the keyboardist for the Temptations (at that moment; the legendary band changes personnel often). I vaguely remember seeing him a couple of nights before he left to tour; it seemed I actually roomed with his clothes. By myself, I would sniff meth all day as I wrote on a laptop for PayPal money. By afternoon, I'd be a bit delirious and start sniffing around on my phone for trouble, and found plenty nearby. I recall one night visiting with a dude down on Broadway downtown, thinking we'd be partying, and the memory hints he was gay and wanted me in bed. Those were the types of situations I'd walk into. After escaping, I checked my phone, and discovered a gal with a current Craigslist ad with a photo of herself from behind in a thong bikini bottom and nothing else. Arms up, holding a lot of yellow-blond hair. This definitely was not a gay trap, I thought. (Long Beach trails only San Francisco for the largest gay populations in the state, more even than West Hollywood). This was the active call girl I would visit with many times the rest of the year. We set a meeting the next day, at a hotel I'd fund over the Memorial Day weekend.

What craziness. She ended up bringing with her a fellow call girl, and we hung out and did meth and I got naked but they didn't and we just hung out for a long time. The rest of the weekend was one long blur. My call girl friend stayed the weekend with me, talking me into placing Craigslist ads for "dates" to come use the room. Once I succeeded, bringing this nerdy married dude from a few towns over. He was over his head in our room, but he did force Roxi to give me a brief blowjob while she rode him. What a new experience laying right next to a naked prostitute and customer as they did it. It didn't seem strange at the time. I was nearing sensory overload.

The weekend got wilder. That we slept in the same bed for two nights without having sex indicates the severity of my condition. She had a rule not to do it with anyone on meth, since the high hinders a guy's ability to finish. A time-conscious business rule. I was on meth the whole time, so that was that. Plus heroin, when her guy visited once and gave me a smoked hit off foil. It put me to sleep, which is probably what my brain craved. The next night I found the room filled with strangers, including some black dude from the neighborhood who knew the call girl. She was talkative and saying she'd offer the guy a "freebie." Freebie, I thought. I paid for the room and got none.

The hotel manager ultimately arrived and ordered everyone out, which I took as meaning me, too. Everyone left, I packed, and walked into the dark toward a bus stop. I walked a few blocks then realized I paid for the night and still had the key. Fuck it, I went back and slept alone there. Returning to the sober living complex the next day, sometime in the afternoon, the house manager was out front talking with a client. It hadn't dawned on me that I should have at least told her I would be away. Some sober living houses require passes, or solid communication with the manager to spend nights elsewhere. She just calmly asked where I was, and I said Simi Valley with my father, and rushed upstairs to lay down and finally get real rest.

June was bad at that eastside sober living house. Not because of the house manager, who was awesome, or her kids or the complex. We got along well, even hanging out together in the living room at times. However during the day I was alone, sniffed ice, and just kept pounding the keyboard for dollars. I was writing online content articles for guys who optimized web-sites for businesses. Dry writing on a range of subjects, all with the goal to fool Google in searches. By then I was good at it. Unfortunately, that holiday weekend with Roxi rattled some brain nerve and it wouldn't stop buzzing. Within weeks I added vodka to the ice, and promptly ran out of money. I wasn't close to making July rent. So I drank even more, and was caught by the manager, who let me stay anyway. Later, she ended up having another client drive me to a psyche ward to clean up. Still, I walked back in. But by Independence Day, days after rent was due, I told the manager my intention to move out. I had to.

Two big bags on my back, I walked a couple of blocks to lie down on the grass of a neighborhood traffic circle, a round park centered by a gazebo, classic Long Beach. I sniffed some meth, then texted an old high school friend who lived on the west side of town not far off the hip Belmont Shore area. He offered a night or two in his condo so I could – what else? – get my shit together. My oldest daughter and son that moment were staying with my father, so they visited and spent the night. It was quite nice. We walked to Belmont Shore, ate at a fancy pizza restaurant, strolled along the waterways under the stars back to the condo, and left early the next morning … for Dad's … without warning him. It was a strange ride, the first time I'd been in a car driven by a daughter. She seemed kind of an angry driver.

Dad was not stoked. He was quiet as I leisured with the kids on the back patio near the pool, and eventually he saw me conversing and looking sober so he let me stay. The kids left and I was assigned to my brother's old room, in the spot where Mom passed in an imported hospital bed. I did fairly well for a spell, writing a lot, and letting Dad drop me off and pick me up from AA meetings. I did manage once to bus and train all the way to Long Beach for meth, and returned home when it was dark. Dad came storming out of the house when I arrived, but it wasn't late and I wasn't drunk. He was clueless about symptoms of meth use. I just had to talk less and get into my room fast and shut the door. He could pick off alcohol intoxication with the best of them, however. For that trip I knew not to drink while scoring.

I kept a routine of consistently sniffing meth while I tapped the laptop. When I first did crystal meth in the early 1990s, it would come in little paper bindles we thought held cocaine. That early ice burned the hell out of your nasal area and tasted foul, unlike coke. But one little line would keep you amped for many hours, sometimes days. While the shit didn't numb your mouth and face like cocaine, this new smelly stuff was ... cheap and powerful. When we had dough and the connect, we'd prefer coke; but eventually more often we sought crystal.

I did it on and off that period, less than cocaine. Then one Easter morning I snorted four little lines while drinking four beers while mowing the lawn, and ended up hyperventilating so badly that my arms went numb. I suspected a stroke, and it alarmed my wife who hustled us to the emergency room. On the way, the numbness spread to my legs and seemed to be worsening. I didn't know I caused it by breathing too fast; the little amount of ice I snorted was that powerful. The nurses sedated me, and I recovered easily. At the time I was a reporter for a newspaper that threatened random drug testing (they never did, in the 30 months I worked there). The next day I sicked out, then had mass anxiety for a while that the episode would be discovered. I didn't often care about such potential trouble, especially in later years, but that time I was nervous.

I pledged to never do meth again, to stick with cocaine. This new meth was just too powerful. I didn't touch crystal again for 24 years. When I finally did, the product wasn't the same, didn't burn the nasal passageway too much, and didn't overly amp like the old stuff. When I did it several days in a row, a nice neurological pathway formed between my frontal and inner brain, zapping pleasure back and forth, establishing a solid highway of addiction. I learned in later years that doing it in the day without alcohol was rather calming, almost like right after that first morning coffee. Maybe I had ADHD, and meth was like Adderall, speed that calmed the brain.

By August 2017 I was in deep shit. Eventually you don't get proper sleep, and the brain malfunctions. You get anxious, paranoid, or psychotic, or all at once. I experienced the latter several times. It happened at Dad's not long after I added vodka to the routine. I was so out of it one afternoon that I *called 911 on myself*, without telling anyone. Dad was shocked when paramedics arrived at the door. I had also posted something of a mayday on Facebook, so friends visited later (thank you, Gina), and my phone and inboxes blew up. First, however, Dad went with me to the ER.

With the doctor present, it was Dad's first experience with me and drugs. Right in front of him I told the doc the level of my meth addiction. He told Dad there is no detox protocol for meth, that it was just three days of sleep and fluids. That's it: let him sleep a few days. Dad nodded in agreement. The next morning though, around 11 a.m., Dad entered my room and said I had to go. Maybe something I said freaked him out, or someone got to him and advised tough love. Regardless of why, it was a decision that came as close as ever to killing me. Within a month.

* * *

I carried the huge backpack several miles, to an Extended Stay hotel to hide out, party alone, and contemplate options. I had some writing money, but couldn't stay in these clean hotels for long. I finally chose to bus and train back to Long Beach, to live who knows where. It was a big *F You* to Dad, and to the world. The LBC had a more comfortable climate, with more services like free daily breakfasts and dinners at a downtown nonprofit (where later I would live for a year). It was not spread out like suburban Simi or the Valley, which forced a lot of walking and bus stop waiting. Apparently I made decent money, writing a ton of articles for a growing window-tinting company with operations in Florida and the L.A. region, which kept my PayPal account healthy. It let me get into $65 per night hotel rooms now and then. The cheap Long Beach hotels almost brought my demise.

The most notorious, for me anyway, was the Club on Lime Street north of Fourth Street. I still get the creeps recalling incidents there. I'd say in a relatively small area of town, there were at least a dozen cheap hotels and motels, most bad, some frightening. At the Club in mid-September, the semi-retired prostitute returned. She agreed to stay with me, Room 12 at the end of the upstairs hall. I'd been in most of the rooms there, but never in 12. Only Room 9 had its own bathroom. The other six rooms upstairs shared a strangely shaped hall bathroom, where at one point the wall narrowed so close to the tub you almost had to turn sideways. Then the elongated room opened up to the toilet, kind of an hourglass shape overall. It was quite the strange and dungy place. People would shower there and then walk in towels down hallways to their room. The rooms were so old they were locked with old-fashioned metal keys, which I learned clients would take to a nearby hardware store to copy. At any time your room could be ransacked, so you had to take anything valuable with you if you stepped away. It was ridiculous, but it was cheap, and Deb loved it. The Indian family that operated it lived downstairs behind the main window, and mostly left everyone alone. It was all sketchy all the time.

The three rooms downstairs seemed less desirable. One faced the management window which made sneaking visitors difficult; and two others were down a hallway where I had several incidents. Downstairs rooms shared their own small bathroom. No one was supposed to have visitors, but everyone did. People often split the $65 and just shared the bed, usually a little bigger than a twin. I slept closely next to some crazies in that place. Homeless chicks, usually older; meth-addled tweakers with face tattoos; really weird gay guys. I shake my head at memories, and for sure I don't remember much.

In Room 12, Deb and I just got into a routine as if we were a traveling couple. We never planned it. We just fell into this groove where mornings we made sure we had (or could get) dope, then I'd slink off to find WiFi to write, usually at a coffee shop. There was a Starbucks down Lime at its south terminus at Ocean Boulevard. It had tall windows and very padded seats and lots of preppy younguns including hot gals. I could spend hours there writing and day-dreaming and drinking, which I did. I "worked" a job in the day and later returned "home" to my lady, with home being a sketchy hotel.

One shift, I downed two pints of vodka while writing, equaling a fifth, or the bigger bottle of liquor similar in size to a common wine bottle. A lot of hard liquor for one daytime sitting. Still, I don't remember being significantly buzzed on the short walk home. Maybe it was the coffee, or my tolerance was reaching stratospheric levels.

I walked into Room 12, and she asked if I wanted a shot, meaning heroin injection. Yes, I said, and she stuck the needle into the backside of my right hand, below the joint point of the index and middle fingers. There's a decently sized vein there, I learned. She injected, and I woke up to see her sitting on the bed opposite me, facing the other way, elbows on knees, smoking. She looked bothered, and exhausted.

I was sitting on the floor, back to a wall, opposite her. "Hey," I said, groggily. She replied without looking at me, "You don't know what happened, do you?" Puzzled and dazed, I replied I did not. "You overdosed." What? "You slumped down from the wall, and when I saw the vodka bottles in your backpack I knew you were in trouble." No one told me alcohol and heroin don't mix. They both lower the heart rate. Together they can dip heart beats per minute so low that you lose consciousness. If you're alone, or with unknowledgeable or unhelpful people, you can die. Basically, opiates can make your heart relax too much. It can be revived; it just needs someone nearby with the ability to think and act.

The day before, I borrowed $20 from a friend working at the laundromat of my post office box (the heavyset cook from the Sally), just so we could eat. (I still owe the cook from the Sally, in fact). My retired prostitute friend explained the mayhem of waking me up.

She reached into my pocket to find the money – thankfully it was there! – and raced down the hall yelling "Tabasco! Tabasco!" for a dealer I'd been buying from for days, at the other end of the hall. She didn't know which room, so she yelled all the way down the hall at every door, until she neared Room 6 at the end. Tabasco answered, a real act of faith. She scored meth, raced back, mixed a dose, loaded a syringe, and stuck the needle into the back of my right hand best she could. Under that vein is hard bone. The needle struck bone and broke, sometimes a big problem. She said luckily she could remove the broken tip, and then opened my mouth to squirt the meth-water mix from the syringe into my mouth. Then she closed my mouth and shook my head to force swallowing. Then she got on to fixing a new batch. This one ready, she just stabbed it into my inside left forearm, or "muscled" it. It doesn't require finding a vein, instead stabbing straight into muscle tissue. It works, but the effect is slower to materialize so it is not preferred by addicts for self-injection. Finally, it was nervous time for her, until my breathing increased. I woke up, saw her across the small room in a light fog, and felt nothing strange. In fact, I felt pretty good. I guess you can feel good coming out of a heroin overdose – because *you're still on heroin.*

After she explained, I sat in quiet disbelief. I knew it was bad. Then I just went about the night, asking few questions but not overly bothered by the fact that, had she chosen to flee the scene, I could have died. It took a couple of years for the incident to shake me enough to really ascertain, and admit to myself, that I was *way sick.*

It served as yet another reminder that this suburban man just didn't have the chops for the streets. Would I ever? Perhaps. I was seeing things never witnessed in nearly five decades of life. Prostitutes, needles, homeless deranged thieves, very hard drugs, and more. And more was coming.

Somewhere in the following days, she walked out. I ended up linking with a gal in Room 11 next door, which started a really weird yet (thankfully) very brief dally. We didn't have sex, though I think I tried in a clumsy brain-fogged way. She said she had a boyfriend in jail, and I have no idea why she let me sleep in her bed with her, in this room packed with crap. She'd camped in there a while. Somehow I left my wallet under the bed when I left.

She bitched at me at the door one day, and the guy next door in Room 10 invited me to stay with him. Still no wallet. I didn't know it at that moment. Not long later, I saw my semi-retired prostitute friend in our old room with a street loser we knew, with my stuffed backpack on the bed. I'd funded our room for more than one day, I realized. She returned for some reason, with that dude, and I vaguely remember seeing her there and walking away. Later, I'd discover some of my favorite surf shorts were missing. Street people will steal anything.

My new host had a spiderweb tattooed on the side of his face. Originally it was done lightly, then someone tried to touch up a darker web on top, and it looked bad. He had left prison not long before, with tattoos everywhere. In his room, we got right to hard dope. He injected me with a dose of meth, and my head spun for hours and I remember only patches of debauchery. He had a snake tattoo winding down his back. All my visual memories are not good. One night, he had a female friend sleep in the bed with him, as I slept on the floor. The next night he brought in a mother *with her small child*, forcing me to sleep in the back of her car parked out front. Waking the next morning, really angry, I exited the car and opened all the doors of her big sedan wide open and left them like that. I stomped up there and darn near kicked down the door to get in. It may have caused some damage to the door jamb and the owner-manager visited to look, and my host convinced him it was fine. Then the host bitched me out. I told him that sleeping out in a car was bullshit since I'd funded the room (or so I guessed). I blew him off, plopped down on the floor, and tried to sleep. He just jumped in the bed and did the same. Later that morn he had me walk the kid's plastic tricycle down to her car, which must have been amusing for the managers of a place disallowing visitors.

The gal of Room 11 was asking around for me, and Spiderweb Face was not divulging. He reported that she had moved downstairs to the undesirable, up-front Room 3. We assumed she needed money to stay longer. The next time she saw my new host, she returned my wallet, saying she just found it after repeated attempts by myself to get into her old room to look. I bought another room for us downstairs, in the infamous Room 5 at the end of that hall. There, the con got weird. I'd already noticed a fairly large handgun sitting on the upper shelf of the closet. My sick mind had shrugged it off. When he started talking weirdly, and kind of pretending to clean the gun while I laid on the bed as far away as possible, facing the other direction and feigning sleep, I got nervous. My paranoia triggered the flight response, and I got up and said I was going to the bathroom down the hall. I went straight outdoors and down the street a block and called 911. I said a guy with a gun was locked in that room, with my stuff trapped inside, and that he might be mentally compromised.

The arriving cops weren't enthusiastic to get involved. There were four of them, maybe five, and they asked whether I was certain it was a gun, and if it was loaded. Yes, it's a gun. I don't know if it was loaded but he seemed to be working on it. One said, "So … You want us to go in there and confront a guy with a possibly loaded gun *so you can retrieve your bag*?" He had a point. They went into the hotel, must have checked in with the manager, and knocked on the door of Room 5. No lights, no response. How the fucker knew they were coming is unknown. The officers came outside, explained the above, and left. I stood in the street in the dark feeling like a moron. Here I was now, locked out, and having to crawl back to get my stuff and away to safety.

Which I did, knocking on the door, and apologizing best I could. He was pissed, rightfully so, asking if I wanted him to return to prison. (Which I did, by the way). He said it was just a BB gun, which I didn't believe but let it go. I just cowed with my head down as we both gathered our stuff since the manager was standing at the door. "You must GO!" he yelled while pointing at me. What a drug-drenched absolute mess.

We walked down Fourth Street toward the laundromat, which was closed indicating the lateness of the situation. He pushed a bike, and said he'd call his father for the night. At the end I said good-bye, turned a corner so he could no longer see me, and ran in a light jog up Alamitos to quickly get space between us. I don't remember where I slept. That concluded an absolutely crazy period of several days where twice I could have died, once by heroin, the other by a meth-crazed gun-toting insane homeless con.

* * *

I somehow managed the rest of September and most of October on the streets. No winter shelter yet, and no plans for anything, really. Just day-to-day wandering. With about a week left before Halloween, I randomly connected by text messaging with an old acquaintance from high school, who I knew better from AA meetings starting in 2009. My friend had a stroke years before and rode an electric sit-down scooter most everywhere, and usually used a cane walking into meetings. His speech was badly garbled, but he shared at every meeting and was super friendly. He always seemed to treat me like I was a former superstar player in Simi High baseball. I wasn't a star, really, but had my name in the local sports section at times. I think it's my unusual last name that people remember, and the fact that I was on the field at all times for two seasons.

He explained that since I last saw him, while riding his scooter across a major intersection, he was struck by a semi-truck and dragged beneath it. With his million-dollar settlement, he bought a house, which happened to have an empty room. I can't remember why the subject even came up. Maybe I posted something publicly on social media that I needed a place to live. Tellingly, no family members or close friends responded. By this point, they were done with my behaviors.

Somehow I convinced the former editor, who'd already that year gotten me into two sober living houses where I lasted not long at all, to fund first month's rent. My new landlord loved sports, with a huge sports-themed living room where we would watch World Series games. I remember watching a game or two there, then being gone for a week in a psyche ward, where I saw Game 5 (which the Houston Astros won in the end over my Dodgers). I saw that from a holding bed at the old Long Beach Community Hospital where I'd stayed previously. Then I didn't see the final games, probably because I was in another psyche ward in the Long Beach area somewhere. Later, I determined I spent 10 days in Long Beach carousing, until my brain could take no more. From a train platform en route to home, I had a passerby call 911. Per usual, I feined suicide and got a ride to a psyche ward. The only thing I remember in Long Beach was cruising around with a couple of gay guys to score meth from a westside park in the middle of the day; and sleeping that night on a cushy black couch abandoned on a Fourth Street sidewalk near Cherry. It was Halloween night, and people walked by constantly. My shut-down brain did not register anything.

Eventually I crawled back to the Simi Valley room, somehow explained where I had been, and my landlord friend seemed to buy it. He'd never seen me drink so he assumed I was sober. That helped keep the heat off. I bullshitted well, and he left me alone to keep using meth and chugging vodka in what in reality was a sober house. The room was big and remodeled and very clean, but the only furniture was a cushy futon as a bed. I never added any other furniture. I stored my little collection of clothes on the high shelf in the closet, where I'd eventually hide big handles of vodka bought at a convenience store that wasn't all that close by. The house was in a poor location for someone with no vehicle, without retail or commercial centers close. I was wicked as the alcohol took over into December. We set a Christmas party for the 8th – my friend always wanted to attract what he called pussy there. He used me to bring some in from our school days. However, in the very early morning of the day of the party, I woke up to a *lot* of blood just sprayed like a hose across the futon and onto the wall. While asleep I sneezed hard and blew an enormous amount of blood from my nose. Somehow in the wee hours I got an ambulance to take me to the ER, where I learned I had a staph infection up the nose or nasal cavity, alarmingly close to my brain. Probably from snorting meth from rolled dollar bills, or from grimy places I'd slept. I didn't make it back until later that night, and upon arriving I discovered the party attracted no one. My landlord and his homeless friend, missing a leg who slept nearby in his van, were alone with a small cooked turkey on the table. I mentioned the staph infection and went to the bathroom. When I came back, the turkey was in the trash. His friend suddenly treated me like I had the plague.

Not long after, I packed and left, knowing again that I couldn't pay rent. The landlord was getting on me for shenanigans, including having visitors in my room for who knows what. I bused and trained back to the newly opened winter shelter in Long Beach, where I'd wander a lot more before finally getting help months later. It was the end of a 15-month run in Hell.

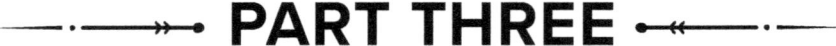

PART THREE

CHAPTER 5

REDGATE 1, 2018

New Day Rising

I always remember March 6 as the day of the fall of the Alamo, my favorite historic event since childhood, nurtured by a father who grew up with Davy Crockett on television in the 1950s. Now it also is the day I first walked into Redgate Memorial Recovery Center in midtown Long Beach, on PCH not far from the Sally. Or, still semi-ghetto, along a stretch of highway sometimes called Hookers Row.

Redgate had a good reputation among recovery dudes I knew who left the Sally on unfriendly terms but then got well at RMRC. As I trudged through the winter shelter again, I called RMRC daily trying to get in. It took a while to finally walk in for detox. The night prior, the receptionist said on the phone, "Drink or do drugs. But don't do heroin." Apparently you had to fail a UA to get in. No problem!

I just happened to have meth on me when, walking around at night aimlessly in the Long Beach Arena parking lot, I ran into a dude carrying a lot of bags. He was completing a trek from New York. He'd just exited the end of the subway line and kept walking toward the water. He was a light-skinned black dude, maybe a bit Caribbean, who ran West in search of a rap career. He said the next stop was the Orange County coast, which I found amusing. It's not Rap Central. It seems he got bad intel. Anyway, he had beer and I had meth, and we hung out right off the water at a marina where he could send videos of himself with docked sailboats and the ocean in the background to friends who doubted he'd reach the Pacific. He was in good spirits and the night went okay, eventually ending at my laundromat with exterior post office boxes, where he spent time washing and drying all his stuff. When done, we walked across a side street and he planted on a wide sidewalk next to a chain link fence blocked with plants at a car service business. It wasn't the best spot, but it would do. He proceeded to spread out all his stuff like it was a campground. All over the sidewalk not far from apartments. I drank one of his beers, and bid adieu. I had Redgate on the mind.

With a small amount of meth remaining, I walked up Alamitos to a favorite spot in front of a long-shuttered cafe, which had a front area bound by metal poles with large tiles on the ground. It was darkened and a little off the busy street where few could see beyond parked cars. It had two big pots where plants once lived, good for peeing. I curled up on my side as usual, resting my head on a forearm. I snorted the rest of the meth and closed my eyes. Maybe it was relief or the meth, but thoughts of no longer having to deal with the streets was calming. A long, drawn-out tour of Hell was officially ending. I slept well.

* * *

Waking with the noise of growing traffic, I stood, stretched some, and began walking up Alamitos toward PCH. It was barely daylight and I had until 8 a.m. to enter Redgate. I'd never been there. It was a decently long walk, maybe six city blocks north, then three long blocks west through Hookers Row. I remember a feeling akin to floating there. The anxiety of waking up and getting on with the task of finding booze wasn't there. Such a relief. Deep in my brain, I felt the walk was to somewhere safe, with people to help. Perhaps it was a symptom of repeated rehab stays. I don't know the reason for the melancholy, because I clearly did not get enough out of previous rehabs. Going into rehab with a good attitude, a feeling of desire, or "wanting it," helps greatly. You can feel inspired, ready for change.

Redgate has a pretty solid reputation around town. I heard the name from many folks in recovery meetings, especially from my punk rock buddy Richard. After a lengthy stay in detox, at least 10 days, I proceeded to recover fairly well. It didn't take long to re-assume my role as a Rehab All-Star. It seems those skills transfer.

I did two stints at Redgate, almost exactly a year apart, through spring 2018 and then end of winter into spring 2019. The first visit lasted three months. Notice how my rehab stays started getting longer? I think I had insurance, through the state, or due to the ACA as explained. Tack on another month for the second stay, as suggested by the program since I returned so quickly. Rehab stints were no longer brief.

The first ended up a waste, since afterward I was directed to a *really bad* "sober" living house, in Compton. That experience lasted just two months and prompted my quick run back to TTC. Redgate 1 and TTC 2 were in 2018. That year was almost as bad as 2017. I had a hellacious run from 2016 to early 2019.

At RMRC, to summarize, it was very good. It didn't take long to realize it may have been my best rehab experience, program-wise. It certainly was welcomed after TTC and the Sally. The Salvation Army ARC was such a drag on my psyche it cannot be overstated. It made me angry at all rehabs, unfairly. Redgate is not large, with indoor hallways like Tarzana, surrounding a decent-sized concrete quad where we smoked and played ping-pong, dominos, and cards.

Counselors and groups were above par. Materials distributed in groups were not outdated, and the program was not overly dependent on the 12 steps, though we had plenty of meetings on site. Redgate had a super impressive alumni organization. We walked on outings frequently, as a group to a store, or the other way to a neighborhood park with a beautiful soccer field. At that park, with a tennis ball, I taught colleagues to play Buns Up from our school days. All that practice at Valley View junior high paid off. What a hoot.

There weren't many troublemakers, few 23-year-old males forced there by mommy, or via nudge from a judge, stubbornly resentful. I don't remember many Rehab All-Stars there. What I did see was a heck of a lot of success and long-term sobriety. Being among graduates was constant: at the center desk near counselors' offices; as volunteer program assistants (PAs); and in the many 12-step meetings most nights. One NA meeting was memorable especially when they gave out chips for clean milestones. I still say the Whiner Chip whenever I see or hear about 18 months clean or sober – something like "We don't have no 18-month chip, Homey!"

My first roommate was James M., a no-doubter Rehab All-Star. Or as I liked to say, I think stolen from Ted Nugent or Blue Oyster Cult, a veteran of many psychic wars. We shared stories of rehabs past, challenges while homeless, near-death experiences, and more. He was a cool roommate with a great sense of humor who was with me the entire first RMRC stay except my final week.

James was such a Rehab All-Star, soon he was elected to our clients' advisory board, kind of the *student council* of rehabs. Where you don't have any true power, but develop ideas for the administration to reject. Actually that wasn't entirely true for Redgate. Sometimes they'd take us up on ideas, like a karaoke night (which Oski dominated, by the way). Soon, James was elected president of the body, at which point he recommended me to join as secretary to take notes. We were community leaders, he even more so than I. We hadn't even been there long. I thought that was rather promising. Maybe my rehab experiences would pay off somehow.

James arrived as a heroin addict, right off the streets, where he lived in a bush somewhere in south L.A. Those types of addicts don't usually last long under those conditions. He walked into Redgate, colleagues said, filthy with a long beard like the guys in ZZ Top. I couldn't imagine it because here was this dude who looked like a clean-cut preppy from the '80s.

When I met him, he had a clean "nice boy's haircut," as my old school bud Mark Akrop would say, showing male pattern hair loss at the part. He was clean-shaven with a huge smile accented by one crooked front tooth protruding a little forward. He was funny and smart. As a Rehab All-Star, he talked often about previous "seasons" – rehab stays – as if we were professional athletes. We started many stories with something like, "One time in band camp (rehab), I ..." Amazing how many similarities we discovered.

James was a workout fiend, and by the end of his months in a little closet of a gym, he looked like a mini bodybuilder. He was a good athlete, too, dominating as goalie in soccer one day, diving all over the place to make stops while I watched from afar as the other goalie. One game ended 0-0, put it that way. No stranger could tell James was a chronic addict, who last lived behind a bush in south No Man's Land. He was so liked by program administrators that, in the final weeks of his program, they gave him a part-time job to work at a hardware store owned by RMRC's parent company, all while living in the inpatient facility. I only saw them do this for one other client, and that guy was 31 and never had a job so they wanted to provide him work experience. James was being fast-tracked, which I took as a positive since he and I were connected nearly all the time.

James had worked in sales before, in what we'd probably consider a mid-level position, and definitely needed no experience with being employed. Still, getting back to working seemed to do wonders for him. Suddenly he seemed all-in on working and trying to be an adult. He left Redgate a week before me, and immediately landed a new job in sales, I think in Orange County. I remember seeing him once more, at an AA meeting at Redgate after I had discharged. He seemed to be kicking tail.

Within months, James disappeared. I heard he returned to heroin and the spot behind the bush. No one knew. Looking back, it sounds like something I'd do. I can't count how many times I relapsed and returned to a previous situation. It's as if we are as addicted to the lifestyle as much as the substances. One time he responded to an email I sent with a single word, and it was the last time I heard from James, much later in 2018.

Redgate is a solid program in a tough neighborhood. There was a decent little park down the street with a soccer field and space for softball. Sometimes we'd go there for groups outdoors, a nice break from being stuck indoors all the time. We'd all sit at picnic tables while a counselor stood and facilitated. Little things like this helped make the program stand out. Those deep into their program time could request passes to leave the facility for a few hours at a time, to visit the library and its computers, to shop, or just goof off. Not the daily freedom of the Sally, but a decent reward for good behavior.

The actual program was delivered well by a solid team of counselors, without question the best since AIA. Which means I went over 60 months without decent institutional programming, 2013 through 2017. Perhaps for RMRC, having the word "memorial" in its name provided incentive to shine. It's like, despite the challenges of this very old facility that looked like a former nursing home, and its location off a sketchy highway stretch, it trudged ahead. The counselors shined, making up for suspicious management. I called it the Little Rehab that Could.

* * *

As usual, memories of the place are dominated by the characters. Joining James and I on the student council was a couple of pretty girls named Jenn and, I think, Kristin. They certainly were BWOC, big women on campus. There was a dorky agitator we'll call Bryan, who was always trying to get Jenn to agree to a date. The looks on her face at these moments were priceless. There was a grouchy hippie-like dude who came from living outdoors near the Forum in Inglewood, a strange place for a white dude to stay homeless. Upon arriving I had no money but still had a nicotine craving. This guy rolled his own smokes and provided me with plenty. I was penniless until RMRC allowed a trip to the county welfare office near Compton so I could sign up for food stamps and what they call general relief, or GR – $220 cash on a debit card monthly. Later, an older guy who had a career in aerospace and knew a lot about the military became a good friend. Within a year he would be sponsoring me there.

Redgate had a very solid core of staffers, including two really friendly maintenance dudes, and PAs who weren't assholes all the time. One in particular, a short cute Asian woman, caught me both stays doing something dumb. It was hilarious after each, because every time she passed me in a hallway she'd squint her eyes and say my name like I was a suspect *for something*. Like "*Keee-thh.*" I'd always laugh. I don't know what it was, but the vibe at Redgate was healthy.

My recovery felt strong at the end of that first Redgate stay, into early June. It would be followed by my first experience where I had to depend on a rehab for help with post-treatment housing, because I didn't have money (or background) to just get an apartment. Fortunately, Redgate owned an apartment complex up the street across PCH, where it sent a number of clients, limited by lack of enough beds. Unfortunately, placement there required some kind of boot-licking, or other political insideness, which I'm no good at. I didn't seem to get much interest in sending me "across the street." Ignoring the reality that there probably just wasn't a bed available, I chalked it up to being opinionated and verbal about most everything. Program administrators dislike smarty-pants clients who just might figure things out, and not always correctly.

Though my own counselor was in charge of placing clients in the Redgate beds, I never felt like a candidate. True, there were only maybe eight beds. But I was a good player with no major infractions who served the student council, and served well. My roommate got right in. When my turn came days later, they said it was all about timing, *if* a bed opens. With only a week remaining my future depended on someone getting ejected or leaving the RMRC sober living complex. Having heard no other options to that point, I was understandably anxious. I felt done with institutional living, surrounded mostly by male addicts. It influenced my decision to accept *any solution offered*.

My counselor steered me to a sober living house in Compton he'd just discovered. Relieved to hopefully have *somewhere* to go and live, I got a pass to go see. I did, at the administrative office of a new intensive outpatient program (IOP) that was *aligned* with the sober living house. The IOP location, with a little room off to the side to host groups, was clean and new-looking inside, located in a crappy neighborhood not far from where they'd show me the house at a later time. The proprietor was a super-sweet young immigrant woman, I think Eastern European, awaiting a permit to administer methadone for opiate addicts. Apparently they secured the lease but plans got bogged by bureaucracy, and to bridge the gap they offered IOP groups for income. Yet another example of a burgeoning big industry. I liked her, but made a near-fatal mistake. I did not insist on visiting the *house*, and walked back to the train to return to my Long Beach rehab. I still remember her saying the house was "nice."

What a crock. It was a complete disaster almost from the moment I saw it. I graduated RMRC, and very quickly discovered that the house was as terrible as anyone could imagine. I relapsed the day after I arrived, and was arrested a day after that for public intoxication somewhere in east Long Beach, after a blackout bus ride. In the process I lost my backpack with a just-purchased used laptop, and somehow dropped a couple hundred bucks from a bank account built only with welfare money, so there wasn't a lot there to begin with. Prior to the aimless bus ride, I spent hours in a blackout drinking with locals on the side of a stand-alone liquor store. I woke up with a near-empty wallet and no backpack. I spent hundreds for … nothing I could remember. After the brief jail stay, to avoid the shithouse of home, I checked into a psyche ward where I stayed a week.

The "sober" living house was a small old suburban abode in what is called East Dominguez Hills, in the classic L.A. tradition of creating new fancy-named mailing districts to separate neighborhoods from the bad reputation of a town name. It's a property-values protection thing. It happens to cities where certain pockets of residents do not want to be associated with their hometown's name. Like Compton, or Panorama City or Canoga Park. In L.A., new communities pop up with names like North Hills or West Hills, sometimes for areas nearly flat as pancakes. Like East Dominguez Hills.

The exterior of my new house was nothing special, maybe a dark mustard yellow. The front lawn grass was yellow and dead and dusty, reminding me of a shaky sober living house in east Simi Valley where I resided for maybe six weeks. Inside the Compton house was a decent-sized living room, with hard-wood flooring, and a small kitchen to the side. I learned immediately that nothing in a refrigerator was respected. My food quickly disappeared. Where the living room and kitchen ended, the circus began. The first room to the right had, I believe, two bunk beds inside, in a dark room with little space. All I could see was clothes hanging all over like curtains. Then there was a bathroom we all shared, especially if the crappier one down our way was full, which was often. Passing the bathroom, you took maybe four steps down into a new room. That little room was where I would live, a top bed on one of three bunks. There were always four or five of us in that room. Through our room was a door to *yet another room* of bunk beds. That's where I started, until I fell off the top bunk while blackout drunk a couple of times and they moved me next door where I stayed the remainder of my stay. The house was packed, almost entirely with black guys, many fresh out of jail. One homeless black guy with difficulty speaking lived in a shed out back. I had a big American Indian in my room, along with a small guy called Shorty, then two others who came and went. Most of my memories are of times shared with Shorty, and to a lesser extent, the Indian. I still say "Just Google it" like the Indian and I joked about for any question asked. Shorty did not know why we found it so funny. I still sometimes say that, with the Indian's inflection in my voice.

Unimaginably awful situations happened. Theft of money right out of my wallet, pulled from my pocket as I napped in the top bunk. Cash gone from my wallet while it sat in my single clothes drawer, again while sleeping. I complained to the house manager and he would just sigh, look down and shake his head, like *I was careless*. Or, *he was sick of it too*. Threats of fights, and I came close twice. One time, Shorty held a pointy shovel out toward my neck, in his mind for protection after I challenged him about my missing money. Later, Shorty got his ass beaten badly by the Indian, in the room with me trapped in a corner watching. They argued, and the little guy broke a plate over the Indian's head, cutting the corner of an eye and infuriating him. Shorty ran out the door, and the Indian found a thick wood table leg to run outside and make chase. I followed outside and saw Shorty in the street looking wide-eyed as the Indian turned to head his way, and I used my arms and body language to get Shorty to *run!* I jumped up and down waving my arms like Carlton Fisk at the end of Game 6 of the 1975 World Series, begging Shorty to *move*! It was insane. Shorty took off, and the Indian ran after him. I texted the house owner and never got a response. The house manager was in the hospital recovering from surgery. There was no structure, and at that time no oversight. The Wild West, only rock 'em-sock 'em brawls instead of shoot-outs. Maybe that was coming.

I stayed not even 60 days. There is so much more I could write about that hellhole, but it's sober living and not a rehab, the focus here. A sequel could be *Sober Living House All-Stars.* Just too much to write about without clouding the rehabs subject. By the end of July 2018, threatened by my new bunk mate just out of county jail and desperate, I posted publicly on Facebook that I *really* needed immediate help to flee Compton. An old high school friend connected me with her brother-in-law, who happened to work for … TTC. From one really bad Wild West town into a semi-bad but at least well-staffed Wild West environment.

I filled a backpack immediately after speaking with him and walked right out of Compton. No notice, no nothing. Good-bye, assholes. That place was called Sherry's Place after a woman who worked for county courts and used her position to pick off jailbirds to funnel to her slum property. She had a system of taking for rent most of your GR money, so all you had to do was get county welfare and you could afford to get in. I just shake my head about it all. Shorty and the Indian called it Sherry's Bug Palace, and a few other clever things.

CHAPTER 6

TTC NO. 2
JULY TO OCTOBER 2018

Meet the New Place, Unlike the Old Place

I walked to the Metro line station in Compton and trained and bused into the Valley. As ordered by my contact, I slept outside TTC right on the concrete porch out front. He advised being there no matter what, and after sunrise they were ready for me. My friend's kindness let me skip a waiting list of a stated 60 days. I never would have survived another week in Compton. You'd figure I'd be grateful, but …

TTC No. 2 was nothing remarkable, yet I stayed quite a while. It felt like another experience where I just didn't have better options, much like the second Sally stay. When you snap out in detox and figure this out, it's not difficult to subconsciously (or even purposely) give up, to go through the motions, eating time and counting days. Not a good place to be mentally.

Physically I was okay, and still maintained friendliness to once again make new friends. As before it didn't take long before I took on special assignments. I was tabbed as meetings coordinator. At the start of this rehab is where I last saw old school friend Ana. Once I had enough time to get passes, I'd visit a government workforce development office to use computers and seek work; or continue a practice that left a permanent dimple on the inside of my left elbow, donating plasma for pay. The former commissary worker mentioned earlier as Shiner from five years prior showed up to a night meeting, and became my sponsor. There were similarities to 2013, namely the big facility. But there also were changes.

First, they moved the smoke pit from a large set-aside area on the asphalt area in the rear, to a tiny square fenced inside the interior quad. Apparently they needed space out back for storage, plus there was a lot of pressure to ban tobacco altogether, but Director Asshole was a smoker and this cage was his gift. He was still there, unfortunately. That cage, and the constant lines waiting for people to finish due to its limited capacity, was a daily drag. The herding feeling was not good for the psyche.

They had shady characters working there. One group presenter, who might have also served as a counselor, was not popular. One day under a chair at a pay telephone I found two $20 bills. Being sober and feeling honest (plus the fact that I noticed a camera above), I walked the cash to the main desk. I told the PAs inside, but this pseudo counselor was there for some reason, and he insisted on "taking care" of it whatever that meant. I handed him the $40. The other staffers gave subtle looks of disgust, so I assumed the unpopular counselor would pocket it. I learned a few years later that the guy was fired for getting too friendly with a female client.

It was a rough detox in the other of TTC's two detox operations. Inside was like the other, but there was no free access to the grassy outdoor quad except for some brief breaks. The indoor rec area, a cage-like indoor box, doubled as the smoke pit. I smoked a lot and listened a lot to a guy who complained constantly about waiting for his Suboxone, then I was finally relieved to the residential side.

The facility looked the same – cushy and colorful low-cut carpeting, wide hallways, barracks-style rooms. But something was different. After briefly talking with my old high school friend Ana, it hit me. This place was *packed* with people. In five short years, Obamacare's monetary incentives came to life at TTC. The population inside increased at least 30%. I was placed in the biggest dorm, seven bunk beds, 14 guys for one bathroom with two toilet stalls and a single-occupant shower. Another dorm the same size was connected with ours. Those poor guys had to walk through our room *just to get to* the door for theirs, a setup similar to my room in Compton only at a much-larger scale. This was where my old school bud Chad stayed in 2013. I was located opposite of where I stayed before, diagonally across the main squarish building, with the large kitchen in between.

My memory hints there were 80 or 90 clients at TTC in 2013; and five years later it was around 140. So many that we were assigned to "groups" for classroom sessions, e.g. you had to remember if you were in Group A or Group B. There were so many clients in the facility that they had to break us up to manage groups. Tack on to that another change: administering the drug Suboxone, mentioned earlier, to help opioid abusers get past withdrawals. While that was the hope, it ended up being just another crutch for those addicts, and they turned into zombies waiting for doses of what also is known as buprenorphine. Big lines would form down a hall for clients to have a Suboxone strip dropped onto their tongue, I think twice a day. After the dropping, clients would have to open their mouth wide and stick out and wiggle their tongue to prove they weren't "cheeking" it, or hiding it to double a dose later for a bigger high. Basically these rehabs were replacing one habit with another, something I didn't understand. This ended up being true at a sober living program in 2024. Guys who were clean from opioids for years due to prison suddenly talked some doctor into prescribing Suboxone, and the sober living program allowed it. Must be another thing from *Rehab Today* magazine. This was new to witness, and it wouldn't go away. Even at Aloha House on Maui, people begging for their Suboxone fix could get it. At a sober living house after my third AH stay, twice I overheard roommates on the phone begging pharmacies for fast Suboxone refills. These were zombies at night. It was pathetic.

Considering the changes I witnessed, I assume there's good money to be made off Suboxone. Reimbursement was probably weaved into an annual ACA update. Which, I would learn later, is fairly typical after mass lobbying by large pharmaceutical and isurance corporations. The whole enterprise is a gigantic taxpayer-supported racket.

Something else at TTC No. 2 was noticeable compared with my first stay: beaten-down staff. The difference in a lady we'll call Sherry was startling.

In 2013, she was a spot group presenter – not a counselor or program assistant, but kind of like a substitute teacher. It felt like when she showed up, she was filling a vacancy, maybe once or twice a week. She was funny, personable, and provided a nice respite compared against stodgy group presenters. In 2013, Sherry was popular and fun and would joke with us, telling the tattooed boys she was from "Hoodlum Hills," a reference to her affluent and mostly white home community of Woodland Hills. She was thin with medium-length golden blond hair, and cute in a way with a big smile. She seemed to enjoy working with us.

By 2018, the joy was gone. The lady who previously was in charge of supervising the entire population (as opposed to The Program, which was overseen by Director Asshole and a special assistant), had passed away. That actually raised flags in my mind because Susan was not old. I eventually wondered if TTC killed her. Having that skinny tall blond lady with the thick New York accent replaced with an evil version of Sherry took time to accept.

Sherry replaced Susan right as TTC hit its stride on the greed train. No longer a fun groups presenter, Sherry now was sheriff in a Wild West town that grew too fast. Under Director Asshole, it seemed she was expected to dole out punishments, and that she did. With so many more clients, far outnumbering personnel, plus a pass system where long-timers could get off campus consistently, the place was ripe for mischief. In my return stay at TTC, I saw everything: fights close to erupting; guys screaming as they carried a stuffed Hefty sack out the back gate; shady counselors who seemed too kind to girls; rumors of shit smuggled inside; threats; and more. It felt like the Wild Wild West, only way more crowded.

As opposed to 2013 when the entire time I had a girlfriend who was actively seeking her own place for us to land, this round I had no such backup. My housing again would depend on the help of a rehab, and the thought all along was to get into a TTC-managed sober living house in the Valley. I was not fond of the concept, but with no other options or ideas I did my time awaiting discharge. Which, just like last time, they couldn't seem to set. It felt purgatorial.

I don't know where three months went, except my dominant memory was always feeling crowded. I had my typical never-subsiding desire to chase tobacco, which meant awaiting money, and for at least the first month I had none. I was living off the $220 monthly from county welfare, and the Compton landlord took the payment at the start of August before I could cancel that arrangement. Going a full month in a rehab without a dime is not fun. Little is worse than living with what felt like a permanent hangover, with no money to at least soothe anxiety with something like nicotine.

I was miserable, and it didn't take long to shift into Rehab All-Star mode. I somehow secured cupfuls of instant coffee, and then instant coffee in bulk, and learned to make it drinkable with just-hot-enough tap water in a plastic soda bottle. Who cares how it tasted? The bump was always needed. My sponsor was a client with me there years before, and took me to night meetings off-site. I started writing my long-promised book based on the Negro Leagues of baseball after Jackie Robinson broke the Major League Baseball color barrier in the 1940s. In fact, I wrote a lot. By hand, filling multiple notepads, all with the intent to transcribe into digital form for editing and expanding (much like for this book).

It was among few things that kept me going. It sure wasn't The Program. The groups were not memorable, the presenters bland and unoriginal, except for an asshole we'll call Jon, a glorified bouncer who was not supervised well. My counselor was still in training, and we never developed a connection like I did with other counselors many times prior and would in the future. It was just an hourlong weekly meeting to endure.

I returned to auto pilot mode. The only comfort was coffee and tobacco, and that meant a never-ending quest for money. Once I was there long enough to get passes approved, I returned to donating plasma in Van Nuys, a trick learned in my journey. I perfected the process and could bring in $300 or more monthly, paid straight onto a debit card, health impacts be damned. Interesting how desperately chasing dollars can be so hurtful for your health.

I always disliked dealing with bureaucracy to get passes approved. My distaste for bureaucracy is a lifelong trait, something in later years had to be suppressed and managed. Another thing I hated was how rehabs punished everyone for the transgressions of a few, or even an individual. My position is punish the culprits or the person, not the entire group. And I was not alone. But TTC applied the opposite tact, with unsurprisingly poor results. For instance, they loved to assign clients to the three-times-a-day kitchen duty, partially to support staff, and also probably to save money, but also to have something to hold over our heads. Few clients volunteered for it. In all honesty, I rarely broke rules so rarely thought about it. They allowed longer passes as a reward for good behavior. I progressed into Phase 4, the very top level except for some long-timers who worked jobs while there, deemed Phase 5. Basically similar to Phase 3 at the Sally. (Notice that below-par rehabs use "phase" systems). I was never late for groups, helped newcomers, and served extra duties like coordinating meetings almost every night. That alone was a huge production, and I didn't mind doing it. Rehab All-Stars know the benefits of leading by example, after all.

Still, I had no program completion date nor housing secured for afterward, no funds saved, and no way really to generate more income. It was yet another situation like the Sally: grind it out and tolerate the best you can because you lack options. The cavalry wasn't coming to save me. No one was, and I knew it, which made it even worse. Most of my friends and family members didn't know where I was; it's no exaggeration to say many assumed I was dead or in jail. My friend Shannon many times said she feared me dead. This, in the end, is the destiny of Rehab All-Stars who are Little Leaguers in real life. It just felt like doing time, with no inspiration, no hope. So I read books and wrote a lot, and looked forward to my next pass and money for plasma that I could exchange for tobacco. It was a long wash-and-rinse cycle, repeated daily and weekly, with no finish line.

One morning a day before I had a pass, in the typical mayhem it takes for 14 men to use a single bathroom and prepare for the pre-breakfast community gathering, we failed to notice a young client still snoozing on the bottom of a bunk next to the door. Typically we nudge each other along to get up and ready and make beds. It's kind of like living in the military this way. I couldn't even see him all the way diagonally across the room. I was a tad behind and was busy looking down working on my bed. I guess we were pulling it close to the daily all-house morning gathering time, and an obnoxious PA walked in and started screaming at us for not waking up in time. The main culprit, a chubby early-20s kid with a nose ring and long curly hair, popped up from his cocoon of sheets and watched as we all were threatened with kitchen duty for a week.

To say we were upset is an understatement. Especially for old-timers like myself who needed time away to seek work and create some sort of future. But TTC being what it was, the next morning two other weasel PAs stormed into the room yelling like middle school yard-duty staff for us to get up and report for morning kitchen duty. It was amusing since most of us planned to blow it off, myself included. I was having none of that bullshit. I blew off the order, ate breakfast, and afterward a veteran roommate convinced me to approach Sherry about our passes. He believed his relationship with her was solid enough that maybe our passes could slide. We approached, she opened the day book showing who was approved for passes that day, and while chewing gum obnoxiously drew lines through our names. Then handed us the book and walked off. She looked like she had aged 10 years since 2013, maybe even more, and it was sad. Not the same person. In my mind I thought, damn, *TTC might kill her, too.*

I waited for the bell to ring. Then I simply walked out the back gate without signing out at the desk per protocol. No one would know I was gone. I had snuck out once in 2013 so I knew it was doable, especially with the huge population greatly outnumbering staff members, most of whom were unhappy and disinterested anyway. Plus, I had a feeling that if caught, I'd be better off homeless in Long Beach anyway. Screw a TTC after-care house. Living in the Valley, especially without a car, was not attractive. The place was a huge suburban nothingness, way spread out, commanding long walks and bus stop waits. My brain longed for a change of scenery.

I got it, thanks to a brain dehydrated of plasma then doused in vodka. I woke up in an ER at a hospital in Encino I didn't know existed (since the Encino hospital I was born in was long gone). When I came to, they weren't helpful, simply kicking me to the streets to ignite yet another odyssey of the absurd: weeks of homelessness, psyche ward visits, plasma donations, an arrest in Simi Valley for public intoxication, freezing nights behind a 7-11 store in Chatsworth, and, finally, a surrendering trek back to the Salvation Army in Long Beach. What would have been a third Sally ARC try lasted only a week, because I'd learned. As soon as I heard the winter shelter was re-opening, I noted the date, and fled.

Eventually I crawled back to Dad's for a surprise Christmas visit, and he reluctantly took me in, after I promised to call Redgate every day until I got back in. Dad drove all the way to Long Beach again the day before my Redgate intake, and I proceeded to use some cash he provided to buy vodka for a last stand. I drank two pints of vodka before sleeping outside the Atlantic Avenue library, to ease anxiety and again fail a UA to get into RMRC.

CHAPTER 7

REDGATE NO. 2, 2019

Lessons Learned and a Men's Program Gift from God

Redgate No. 2 began with detox, then assignment to the same counselor, who almost immediately said something I remember and repeat to this day: "To maintain recovery, you have to make it *the top priority*. The No. 1 most-important thing, before the girl, the house, the car, the job ... before *everything*." I returned to my new room and bed kind of pissed. *Fuck that guy*, was the thought as I stared at the ceiling and stewed. But in the days following lying in that bed, I had a mental epiphany. My counselor was right. I thought, Holy shit, *I'm very sick*. I really am, and I need serious help. I really have a serious mental illness. That memory remains to this day and the moment helped launch a pretty solid rehab stay that kicked off about 16 months of sobriety. It was a long lesson on acceptance.

* * *

My counselor and I agreed that for this revisit I should stay longer, or four months instead of three. Aside from that, the only element different from the year before was the characters. During my first visit the cast was pretty solid, with James, Jennifer, et al. When I returned, it was even more ... memorable.

Where to start? There's Sara, the single mom who remains a friend today. She became close with someone who on Facebook calls herself Tina Pajamas. Those two alone were worth many laughs. There was a big black former high school football player who followed me over from detox and ended up being my roommate; Cerissa who also remains a friend today who is fighting a disability diagnosed after she sobered at 37; a returnee from Catalina who was with me the year before; a friendly relatively soft-spoken Latino who ended up being elected student council president near the end of my program which for reasons I can't remember got way political. There was a guy calling himself Harris, who hardly spoke English but enrolled to please his wife after a DUI; Oski, a rock band singer fiercely committed to recovery; and our mutual sidekick, Nolan.

Perhaps the hardest I have ever laughed was in a group one day sitting next to Cerissa against a wall, while a group of clients sat circled in the center-room. I think it was a makeup session for us since we were off to the side and not really participants in the session. I loved opportunities to hang with Cerissa, as she was really cute and super friendly. Well, early in the meeting, Harris walked in looking confused, so he grabbed a chair against the wall opposite us and sat. This triggered a running commentary by me to Cerissa, about what Harris was thinking just by the looks on his face, since he didn't understand English. We thought for sure he was sitting in by accident. It looked like he'd walked by, saw the group in session, and jumped in believing he belonged there and didn't want to get in trouble. Right away, his worried expressions indicated he didn't know why he was there, or the topic.

After a while, all us against the walls started to fade out, as rehab clients are prone to do if not truly engaged with group discussions. I looked over at Harris and clearly he was daydreaming, glazed eyes stuck on a spot on the ceiling. I continued the running dialogue telling Cerissa what Harris was thinking, and both of us struggled mightily to not burst out laughing. Then, a question arose in group that triggered a reaction, and I blurted out, "Ask Harris!" At which point the guy nearly jumped out of his chair, eyes wide with surprise. Not only was he caught daydreaming, but he also had no idea what the discussion point was. He just sat there frozen until someone in the group began talking to save him. I laughed inside so hard, I thought I cracked a rib. I know Cerissa struggled, too.

Sara was a solid source of entertainment, since she sure could dish out insults on the equal with me. She was early-30s, super cute, from an Arab family so she couldn't stand seeing feet (which I still don't get), and let's just say she was big-boned. Curvy, that is. She was another mom trying to get her kids back from the government by doing rehab. I can only imagine how hard that must be.

In Redgate, we spent a lot of time standing in a hallway line waiting for meds, some in the morning, but especially at night. This was an opportunity for guys and gals to mingle, because there wasn't much they could do about it, plus the place was rather lax on that rule anyway unless touching was witnessed or suspected. So Sara, Tina, and I bantered every night. Especially Sara, who would respond to my wise cracks by pretending I had a crush on her, which she assumed was a reason I picked on her often. I especially was fond of an incident in a group where the host had us talking about memories of smoking pot, or something triggering like that, and Sara suddenly stood and blurted out, "That's it! I'm outta here!" and stormed out the door. I would do imitations in the hallway in med lines, and still chuckle at the memory. The jabbing went on for some time, and since she would do the *"Aw, you love me"* act out loud, sometimes PAs or staffers would walk by and hear things, and it made me nervous that we might be singled out. Not only did I not want trouble, I was like 20 years her elder. I want to avoid *that* conversation with staff. Sara hated her counselor, and I did a good imitation of that person which Sara appreciated. "Lights out," the counselor would announce over the intercom some nights. "Lights *OUT!*" with oomph. Every time. Like most counselors there, she knew I was doing the impersonation. I said while entering most groups, "Who got da sign-in sheet?" That counselor for sure knew I was doing it.

After leaving there, Sara, Tina, and I became good friends on Facebook. All of us would relapse here or there, and they would sometimes hit me up for cash during rough spells, and I obliged. I knew how they felt and the sorrow with another relapse. It seemed Tina was bouncing all over the most redneck areas on the West Coast, starting near Palm Springs in the 909 area code, and at one point landing somewhere in Oregon, jobless and carless, before meandering back down to Southern California. I think at one point she ended up in or near the same town Josh from AIA wound up. Being stuck in The 909 didn't sound fun.

For the first half or more of the stay, Oski was a primary character. A veteran of the L.A. rock scene, alcohol and especially meth finally nudged him to Redgate, his very first rehab. He would say with confidence that it would be his *only* rehab, and ended up true to his word. He maintained the rock star persona, black hair greased back, jeans, black boots and all. He was a cool cat and much well-respected, ultimately getting elected student council president. I remember in one such meeting, some other client stood at the door and barked at him about something, which was annoying. Oski finally had enough and yelled something like, "That's it! Meet me in the office!" as he stood and chased her down the hall. We all just sat there, student councilors without their leader, the rest of clients spread out among the plastic seats, boys on one side, girls on the other. Oski finally returned, apologized for the outburst, and went right back to where he left off.

Then there was Nolan. I gave him about as much shit as I did to Sara. He was young and cocky and wore these white gym socks with colored stripes at their tops a la the 1970s, and he wore them with pride, like it was *in*. Nolan thought he was way cool, like beyond most of the rest of us. Oski rode him pretty hard for that, too. (To his credit, Nolan did a spot-on impersonation of Oski walking into a meal line). Nolan is a smart, good guy and we spent plenty of time together surviving 12-step meetings. Probably my biggest memory of Nolan was when he broke my room window literally a foot from my head, with a soccer ball he was kicking hard in the quad against the wall next to my room. Scared the hell out of me, and I ran to the quad door to yell at him harshly, with counselor Brittany standing out there wide-eyed because no one had seen me livid like that. It would be a few years later that I accepted the fact that I have anger issues. That situation sucked because I had just days remaining and they forced us to move to a new room. It was an unfortunate ending to Redgate No. 1 right before moving on to the Compton catastrophe.

* * *

Not very deep into Redgate No. 2, and with Compton fresh on my mind, I decided to take my future into my own hands. Once settled in, I called a hospital volunteer I met in an ER a few months prior. We chatted while he cleaned around my hospital bed, and he saw my homeless bags and mentioned Christian Outreach in Action, a nonprofit that provided cooked meals twice day down the road. I was familiar with COA because I'd eaten there many times. Jimmy explained its men's program, which offered housing in exchange for volunteer hours. I took his number and actually saved it. Somehow along the journey I didn't lose the little paper slip, and remembered our conversation. It was another God moment in the odyssey.

At around two-and-a-half months into the 120-day stay, I called Jimmy, who linked me with a call with COA's director. Then I got standard passes to leave campus to interview with her and the nonprofit's president of the board, a wise old gentleman who owned an auto dealership in town. Super nice, solidly Christian folks, which did not bother me. I was a Salvation Army veteran who knew the Bible and needed salvation, after all.

Landing with the same counselor who'd sent me to Compton, I was clear indicating there was absolutely no way I would return to that. Weeks later I explained what I heard about COA. Ultimately COA offered me a test program: volunteer 30 hours over a 30-day period to qualify for the men's program. It was a miracle they had a bed open, since they had only seven beds total – four right next to the main church in a small structure built a hundred years earlier for the pastor and his family. The program also owned an apartment up off PCH in the vicinity of Redgate, in the semi-ghetto Hookers Row area. The counselor sure balked when told I needed a lot of passes to get to the 30 days, but I carefully explained how I could work it in without missing any groups or program, so he reluctantly agreed. The pass system was rather complicated with forms in a binder at the center desk, and to avoid that, the counselor arranged for a running pass, allowing me to leave a lot without having to submit a new request for each one. The volunteers at the center desk got used to me after a while and it worked out fine.

Not a rehab, the COA men's program was a sober living-like operation that had random pee tests, an off-site manager who visited periodically, and side projects that engaged you with churches or other volunteers to help the needy. Finishing Redgate, I moved into the tiny house on Linden Avenue at Third Street, and proceeded to kick ass, ultimately reaching well past a year sober before the next slip. I loved living and working at COA. Search YouTube for Christian Outreach in Action and you can see several videos hosted by me, a couple long-form ones explaining COA, many others showing how we continued to serve the homeless early in the pandemic. My main job, though, was selling donated items online for cash for COA. I was good at it, and had a super short commute. I absolutely loved my time at COA and miss all my friends and colleagues there. I met so many wonderful people.

At the end of 2019, another God-shot chance surfaced, and it wound up changing my life dramatically. A lot of really good things happened from mid-December into the first months of 2020, which as everyone knows became a year remarkably different than any other. My second consecutive girlfriend named Karen was a classmate who graduated with me at Simi Valley High School in 1984. We had become friends on Facebook months before, but I confused her for another blond I befriended there (who happened to be in recovery, the reason we connected). For about three months, when I saw Karen's face in a tiny bio image, I thought she was someone else, who I didn't know well so I never reached out.

Finally one day, on a Sunday bus ride to another plasma donation before Christmas, I scrolled Facebook on my phone and again ran across Karen's little profile photo. For whatever reason – divine intervention? – I clicked on the photo for a closer look. This enlarged the profile pic, which triggered a memory: *Is that the cute, super friendly and kind of flirty little blond from school?*

I messaged her to ask. She was, after all, already a friend on the app. She confirmed, we had a fun little flirty convo before they sucked out my plasma, and we set a meetup for mid-week. By week's end we were dating. Fate would prove wonderful, challenging, educational, fruitful, and sometimes frustrating – all in one little package. I was high with happiness.

* * *

We had a wonderful Christmas and holiday season. She took me to Simi to spend Christmas Eve first with Dad, and then at her mother's place not far away. Her mother suffered from Alzheimer's *and* Parkinson's, a tough road for any family. I learned Karen had lived within a mile of me all through secondary schools. Amazing that we reconnected after not seeing each other for 35 years, since the last day of high school, in fact.

Only a few weeks later, days into the year 2020, I fell extremely ill. For days I couldn't leave my bed. It was an extreme challenge to walk to the bathroom to relieve myself, or even reach the kitchen for a bite to eat. And this was not a big place; we're talking only a few steps needed. Yet I just didn't have the energy. After many days, Karen took me to the ER due to very shallow breathing. After about an hour of sucking oxygen, the hospital discharged me. When I asked about the cause, they shrugged it off, and said only, "Some weird virus." Go figure. Looking back, Covid-19 had been in the news at least a month by then. That an American hospital was not watching for it says something about our health care system. There was some distinct disconnect between the local providers and state and national agencies we trusted to monitor that stuff. The "health experts" seemed asleep at the switch.

I barely recovered enough by the end of January to go with Karen to Maui, Hawaii, where she owned two condos. For 10 days I had the best tour guide, and fell in love with Maui. Still, on the very last day, we broke up. I spent a sad quiet ride to the airport, then a very lonely flight back, as she stayed on island to finish up some business. On the flight I had two beers, which didn't have an impact immediately but in just a few months would get troublesome. The wire was tripped, but it took some time for the monster to re-engage.

We reconciled enough to spend Valentine's Day evening together over pizza and sodas in Belmont Shore, but leaving her car at night when she dropped me back at COA was awkward. I guess offering only a hug good-bye was not enough. Who knew? This forewarned of relationship struggles to come. I'll be honest, and I've said this to people many times while sober over the years: I absolutely suck at relationships. That's a study for a psychoanalyst for another time. I can say as of this writing I'm a little better, mainly because I improved my ability to feel empathy, and have patience. But I still suck.

We became a couple again, and then the pandemic and lockdowns hit. All the national news was alarming and confusing. Rules seemed to change every day. Wash your hands! No, not just that, now do this! Finally, they just closed everything down and tried to lock us away. Not the best situation for developing a romantic relationship. We felt cursed.

We persevered, wearing paper masks as we toured empty streets with closed businesses boarded up, taking a lot of photos of things we figured we'd never see again. I remember going to the very top of Signal Hill, a landmark kind of looming over everything in the mostly flat coastal region, and marveling at what we saw. There were huge oil tankers lined up as far as we could see. Due to the threat of spreading the virus, and the fact that the ports stopped accepting oil since no one was driving cars and demand evaporated, tankers that had been on the open seas for months were stranded offshore. Long Beach residents are used to seeing a single tanker slowly coming to port. To see a lot of them anchored all the way to the horizon was extraordinary.

Something else stood out, and triggered suspicion in my journalist mind. The news repeated ad nauseum that the biggest issue was overwhelming hospitals. So much, in fact, that they made a big deal when a former Navy ship was painted all white, filled with hospital beds, and docked in New York City. It was quite the visual. The problem was, they weren't needed. During the first two months of the lockdown, Karen took me to the hospital twice. The emergency rooms were not overwhelmed. Up on Signal Hill, we could clearly see the big white West Coast version of the floating ambulance, docked right next to the Queen Mary. It was a very brief docking. That ship was gone within days. I don't recall a single bed being used, for the entire huge L.A. region. How peculiar.

Karen began complaining that I was working closely with homeless individuals, who didn't take precautions like wearing masks or staying six feet apart. For a while she pressured me to ask the program to stay with her for a couple of weeks, to quarantine and stay away from potential infection. But a strange thing was happening. No homeless individuals I knew got sick. Not one. The guys in my house, who'd been working among the homeless for years, were not surprised. They said houseless individuals have the strongest immune systems due to constantly being among unclean environments. It made sense. Yet, the news never mentioned anything about it, and soon government medical "experts" poo-poo'd the whole natural immunity thing, and went straight into the Great Vaccine Race. A lot did not check out, and I said so, to Karen verbally, and online a lot on social media.

In my mind, a virus that infected less than 2% of the population, and among those infected, killed less than 2%, was not cause to shut down the national (and global) economy. In the end, everything I suspected and predicted – that the virus was man-made, a lab error let it escape, the news media massively exaggerated and catastrophized everything, and we couldn't trust the infection and death numbers – proved true. But it would be a few years for the truth to bubble out. Meanwhile, this national disaster triggered my news and government curiosity, which grew frustration and anxiety. It was not a good situation for trying to stay sober, and I should have known. Yet I couldn't let it go. I'd get mad arguing with people online, and upset at city or state officials for their decisions. I don't want to delve too much into the Covid-19 fiasco; let's just say by early May, I was drinking.

It was the same story: sneaking a vodka shot here or there, skipping booze for days sometimes, but over-doing it others. Karen grew up in a Mormon family and was unfamiliar with alcoholics, and did she ever get a crash course. Very soon, she noticed. We trudged ahead the best we could, until I landed at her condo for several days, where I talked her into letting me detox while she monitored. Not long after, the men's program manager called to check in. He was homebound by doctor's order due to health matters. I confessed that I hadn't been sleeping at the COA house. It was a no-no, he said, that could get me kicked out. After a brief discussion with Karen, I let them know I was moving in with her. My year at COA, a wonderful era, was ending.

I lived in that Long Beach condo just a few weeks, before she again talked me into visiting Maui, where her vacation rental condo sat empty due to Hawaii's strict quarantine rules. We flew out the afternoon of May 31, right about the time a parade organized to protest the George Floyd police killing began in Long Beach. By the time we landed, got thoroughly screened by airport and island police, and walked into the studio condo, our hometown was ablaze and in a state of lawless mayhem. We arrived the same day Long Beach was victimized, along with Santa Monica, with what proved to be planned riots of looters and vandals. It was so sad and unbelievable. I wouldn't leave the island for two years. I did not stay sober that entire time. Within five weeks I drank, and by the end of July, Karen found a rehab up the huge Haleakala dormant volcano.

Back to the Long Beach relapse that got me out of COA. It was late April 2020 when I relapsed. Not full-bore at first, but a few drinks here or there, spread out. It was a slow kill, kind of like my first relapse from June 2010 to my first rehab in February 2012. At least the previous relapse experience taught me where this would take me. I was cognizant of bad trouble brewing. Again, Karen was unfamiliar with alcoholism, but learned as we went along. By mid-year she would be an expert. Today, I'd say she has a Ph.D in recovery.

The relapse went on and off through May, and I spent many nights at her place, unbeknownst to the COA staff as explained. It didn't take much to move straight down Third Street into her place, but I kept volunteering at COA just two miles away. Besides writing content for websites for cash, I didn't have much to do. The government's pandemic payments were more than I needed. I ended up punting $500 a month to Karen, which she appreciated since suddenly her rental condo income disappeared. The pandemic response was mishandled and hurt a lot of Americans, too often overzealously or even unnecessarily. Long Beach became a ghost town. We watched huge passenger ocean liners, dwarfing the Queen Mary in size, anchored on a small off-shore oil platform disguised as an island, waiting to unload passengers. The government wouldn't let them. Everyone was crazy nuts about the virus. Eventually the liners disappeared. Where they went, who knows? Their docking spot remained empty.

We lived in a subregion with Long Beach and neighboring San Pedro, each with ports that when combined placed it second-busiest in the nation after New York. The big difference is, New York did not take most of its cargo directly from China, where the virus originated. Long Beach-Los Angeles did. Basically, every shipment from China arriving to feed the Greater Los Angeles Area passed near us daily.

Karen made a living renting those condos on Maui – one long-term, or for at least six months at a time, but especially the other which was deemed short-term which meant more income (with tourism). At that moment they sat empty. We could hardly exercise, with gyms closed and passersby frowning on us walking around in the (gasp!) open air taking free vitamin D from the sun. God forbid anyone enjoy themselves alone, away from anyone else. Some unelected God-assuming creature decided to make the country the NFL – No Fun League. Once, sitting together on a huge swath of sand, with no one within 100 feet, a lifeguard approached and forced us to put on paper surgical masks. He was embarrassed, but do it he did. It was insanity.

By the end of May it struck Karen: let's get out of here and away from the homeless and ports. Let's go to Maui where there are no visitors, and a state-mandated 14-day quarantine rule left vacation rentals empty, with no end date in sight. We won't again have an opportunity to see towns like Kihei completely devoid of tourists and traffic, she said. It didn't take much convincing. Off we went to Maui on May 31. The stay was planned for a month. I did not step foot again in California for over two years. Hawaii's governor kept extending the quarantine, and since both of us worked off laptops, we pushed out our return flight each time. This continued every month through the year.

Sometime in early July, frustrated with being stuck in a studio apartment with someone who rarely rests, and who had the opposite sleep pattern, I relapsed. She was able to get me out of the first wave of relapse, but not the second. By month's end she drove me up the mountain to leave me at Aloha House, a substance abuse treatment center. All that work for a year with COA, wasted.

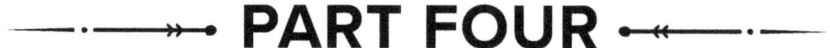

PART FOUR

CHAPTER 8

ALOHA HOUSE
MAUI, 2020 TO 2025

Accidental New State

After a brief stay in a little detox house, I discovered a special little treatment program in the Upcountry region of Maui, on a lush rolling property with ocean views. Of course it did not take long to shift into Rehab All-Star mode, never missing group or even being late, taking on multiple chores, the works. They didn't have a student council-like group for clients, or I could have ended up with that, too.

I got to experience rehab during a pandemic lockdown. Due to the virus, many extracurricular activities I enjoyed in later stays were not happening. No weekly kickball or beach trip. Just outdoor volleyball on a hard dirt court pocked with embedded rocks with a sagging net. I never was healthy enough to play. Instead, I walked for cardio back and forth up a long parking lot driveway while everyone played volleyball.

Program-wise, it was similar to Redgate. So I experienced two treatment centers in a row with above-average recovery programming. The skilled counselors cared, and I was assigned a superb one. He was heavily spiritual, and spot-on with regard to the 12 steps, and other recovery-related guidance.

What marked this rehab stay, my 10th, was the loss of my wallet beforehand. Maui police found it and sent a letter ordering to retrieve it by Sept. 19, or it would be destroyed (their word). I told the counselor, who submitted a transportation request, which the transportation guy rejected because he said Kihei was too far away. After relaying this to my counselor, without any movement, plus his seeming disinterest regarding post-treatment housing into the fifth week of program, my anxiety grew unbearable. In my mind, I had to set a deadline to get to Kihei and the wallet no matter what. I set waiting until Sept. 18, a day before the MPD's date to toss the wallet. I couldn't bear losing my identification card, which is not easy to get in Hawaii, nor my bank debit card. I had some money on that card, for some reason, probably pandemic relief funding. I was itching to spend some. In short, weeks in and feeling good again, I was prone to an excuse to flee Aloha House.

They obliged with inaction on transport, so with all my clothes packed, I walked into the office at 6 a.m. on the 18th, gathered my meds and other property, and walked down Baldwin Avenue several miles to reach Paia and a bus stop. A couple of bus rides later I was in Kihei, ready for a night on the streets to allow me to walk into the police station early. The PD's property folks were only scheduled there a few hours on Wednesdays, but Karen visited in early afternoon before, and they had left. It's a small island with probably a single property team, which I assumed roved around. I could see mornings being slow and them leaving early to serve another office, or just screw off. I knew Maui government workers well enough already. My plan was to walk in right when the doors opened. It worked.

Wallet in hand, I bought a week at the closest hotel, Maui Coast. I don't remember much of my stay there, except eating at a restaurant on its property right on Kihei Road, and a memory that for some reason they wanted me gone. Even though the hotel was really empty due to the quarantine order, it was expensive. I moved on to a week on the other side of the island, north to Kahului. The relapse worsened and dragged on.

Ultimately, Karen took me back and baby-sat my sorry ass until I could get into a sober living house, which took until January 2021. I was there seven months before relapsing and starting the second Aloha House stint, almost exactly a year after my first stay. My old counselor was there, but I was assigned a new counselor, a woman who a year prior was a P.A. She was fresh out of training and seemed overwhelmed, as if forced into it. On a small island, the talent pool is limited. You run across interesting work situations, like trying out a program assistant as counselor, a position typically requiring an education certificate. I had mercy and tried to be the best client possible. My thought was to stay sober afterward for her, and *out of spite* for my previous counselor. I'd developed a decent resentment, which would eventually vanish when I realized that relapse was all on me (and the transportation coordinator, if anyone else). Anyway, as if anyone would care that a rookie counselor did what no one else could: fix Keith. They had plenty of clients to think about. Plus, I was not close to being fixed.

* * *

By this time, any astute AA member could recognize a pattern in my rehab failures. I would let a resentment burn, until it was red hot, and then use it as an excuse to leave program and drink. Both TTC stays ended that way. I subconsciously sabotaged Sally No. 2 by drinking nights. There, it got down to a mindset that I had only a month to go, with little money and great apprehension about going back into a sober living house. Remember that move from a three-bed to a big seven-bed room? Poor me, didn't get promoted to that two-bed room. Woe is me, might as well drink.

At Aloha House No. 2, my Rehab All-Star instincts kicked in. I stayed ahead of the writing required, didn't ask much from my counselor, and played a little volleyball and even kickball when my joints allowed. You start to forget atrocities of the previous relapse, then reminders surface.

Once while leaving Baldwin Beach to end a weekly excursion, we walked past a pasty white, heavy-set guy with a big bald head and pockmarked shoulders. He was standing at his car, driver's side door open, talking to himself, maybe dancing lightly to music from his car stereo. I could hear him saying something to other clients about Aloha House, as if he knew where we came from. As I neared, I recognized him. A housemate at my sober living house, recently discharged, and now high as a kite in a public beach parking lot before noon. Well, Maui locals don't take kindly to white guys high in public. We had to keep one among our group from killing Pasty Man.

It dawned on me that resentment for that former housemate, coupled with my usual anxiety about making rent, knocked me out of that solid sober living house situation. I learned later that the guy was kicked out of our house only a week after I left. That happens at rehabs and sober living houses sometimes. One guy crashes, and starts a domino effect on others. Often it's because that one guy smuggled in dope, and slowly turned other dudes onto it. They always get caught. Every reputable place has drug or alcohol screens regularly, plus they are run by addicts in recovery who easily notice traits of someone blocked up. Honestly, why anyone would want to do drugs while in a rehab or sober living environment is beyond me. Sure, I drank at some, but only later at night, before bed, in my room alone while reading. Not walking around engaging with others, and especially not hard drugs which can make you act weird.

I learned that not long after we saw Pasty Man, he was in jail, with no release imminent. While he was with me in that house, he already was out on bail for "attempted homicide on a peace officer," which he blew off as an accident where he simply let off a car's parking brake and his car rolled too close to a cop. While awaiting trial for that, he tacked on a whole bunch of new charges, and made headlines.

This guy led police on a medium-speed chase all over the island in spectacular fashion, running through central Maui neighborhoods where I'd lived, all the way to Paia on the north shore, then all the way south through suburban Kihei and affluent Wailea. The latter was a bad idea, since that road dead-ends not far beyond, at Makena. During the run his car side-swiped a parked vehicle, and *struck a jogger*. Which all seems amusing since the policy for police here is not to make chase, hence my wording "medi-um-speed." There's no high-speed police chases on Maui, and unfortunately savvy law-breakers know it. The cops will just patiently wait you out. What could you do? Roll onto a ferry and escape to … another island with nowhere to hide? Dumb criminals. He finally was trapped at the end of the road in Makena and caught. The news reports ran his mugshot and emphasized he'd been arrested 70 times previously. Ouch.

When I returned to that sober living house, the house manager (The Chopper mentioned in the Foreword) said he saw our friend at the hospital, handcuffed in a wheelchair, wearing jail orange. The jail took him there for medical attention. He said to my house manager, "I'll be getting out soon." Chopper said nothing but told me later his thought was, "Yeah, right. *You're not getting out.*" Haha!

* * *

My first stay at Aloha House was five weeks, into September 2020. The second visit was almost exactly a year later, maybe starting a tad later like mid-August. From that point, I stayed sober the longest period yet, 23 months deep into July 2023. The relapse commenced just before the historic Maui fires of Aug. 8, 2023. The disaster did not cause the relapse; that seed was already germinating. The fires and mayhem and sadness afterward nurtured and prolonged my misery. I didn't really snap out of it until February 2024. That June, with almost four months sober after a mini-relapse, I decided it was a good idea to attend a 40-year high school reunion on the mainland. That started a relapse that continued when I returned, and in short order drove me right back up to Aloha House for a third stay. After that, back in that same sober living program, in exactly the same bed. *Ground Hog Day* revisited.

Aloha House is the best rehab I've experienced. The campus alone, up the slopes of the huge volcano mountain, is dreamy. It was cooler and more shaded than the towns below. The views from up there could be spectacular, the cool breezes splendid. The property was nicely arranged in smallish separate buildings spread over a gently rolling hill. It was lush, very green, and frankly too nice to be *just a rehab*. Detox was in a single building right up front, next to an eight-bed mental health hold I never lived in. Residential folks were forbidden to linger near the mental health hold, and there were rules just to revisit the detox and see a nurse, who when on duty was the medical eye for the entire property. Nearby was men's Dorm B, an elongated barracks-style cabin sleeping 14 in two-bed rooms. Next to it uphill was an old, elevated building that served as kitchen, with a large outdoor deck with nice views for dining. Across from it, in a central spot, was the main office and front desk, with a small women's dorm inside just down a hallway. Down a hall the other way were counselors' offices, a small meeting room, and washer-dryer setup.

Further uphill, next to the office was a large classroom with administrative offices off to the side, a place where we spent a lot of time sitting in group sessions. The last building up the hill was Dorm A, a resort cabin-like building with a large living room and multiple rooms with 16 beds total. This was the home of veteran rehabbers, or those who'd been there a week or two and were not known or expected to cause trouble. Newbies and troublemakers were destined for Dorm B. For my third Aloha House stay I rejected an offer to move to Dorm A, to remain with a cool young colleague named Thomas.

Back up front, off to the side of detox and down a slope was a dirt volleyball court, where we spent a lot of afternoons bashing the ball jungle-style back and forth over a drooping net. The whole property was at the end of a curvy road, where we sometimes would be led on walks. The setting certainly was awesome, but it wasn't the primary reason the place was special. The programming was similar to the above-par schooling at Redgate. Solid and up-to-date materials, excellent counselors and group facilitators, plenty of rec time and a weekly beach trip, and huge portions of very good meals three times a day. Then there were the characters, colleagues filled with aloha. Friendliest fellows and gals I ever spent rehab time with.

* * *

I entered Aloha House No. 1 as a Rehab All-Star. This time, though, my emotions overwhelmed me, and I missed Karen badly. My thoughts ran wild. I'm living in what they call paradise, so why even *consider* drinking?

As always, I kept asking myself what happened. It was a serious period of self-reflection. I was not getting any younger, and these rehab stays were getting old. Now, my relapses were almost always brief, usually three weeks. I believe this is because my liver stopped processing alcohol well. It was like an old stereo receiver that had its day but now due to mass over-use was merely functional, with less power or clarity, like any gadget or appliance that ages. Sure, it still works, but … Glitches. The experience of being drunk had changed dramatically and at least some of it had to do with physical damage from the poisons.

Karen drank a little, but rarely, and never close to the volumes I'd consume. She had no experience with addiction at this level; and alcoholics in particular can be unpredictable. She would not be the only person shocked by my behavior when my blood-alcohol content neared or exceeded 0.20%. Plus, with my first relapse with her in April-May 2020, she got to experience detox days when I needed monitoring for days. She proved a good learner who helped in each of my Maui relapses. Sadly, our relationship as lovers did not recover. She witnessed too much insanity and had too many bad memories. It would take some time, but eventually we settled in as best friends. We know we wouldn't last as a couple, and that's fine for us both. As long as we can still hang out and have fun and truly experience life, I'm happy.

* * *

It didn't take long to realize Aloha House was a good program. Sure, it had its moments, like when an over-aggressive PA would get anal with the rules. Anal meaning "personality traits associated with a fixation … such as excessive orderliness or stubbornness." Yeah, several of those early Aloha House PAs were anal. Fortunately, the program fixed it by 2024. Until then, I'd have my usual rebel-against-dumb-rules temper tantrum now and again, but they were brief and uneventful. My rebellious tendencies were fading, whether naturally from old age, or maybe years of recovery programming. I no longer devised big revenge plots in my head. The views, climate, aloha, and vibe made it hard to get upset, and especially to remain that way.

I had an excellent counselor, rather hard-lined, but I knew that's what was needed at the moment. He knew the Steps intimately, probed with the right questions, and sprinkled in enough spirituality (God, in his case) to help, without going overboard which tends to turn me off. He gave homework after pretty much all of our meetings, I did a lot of writing, and met all deadlines as usual. I was, after all, a Rehab All-Star. Acing homework was automatic.

I knew what I *was not*, and that was not recovered. I would way too easily let my character defects lead to trouble. I was unable to identify situations which made a defect or two bubble to the surface, or apply tools or tactics to put out fires. Hence, the go-get-wallet excuse to leave the program early. Or, getting mad at TTC for a pass being canceled. There are more examples and none of the experiences ended well.

* * *

The involvement by Karen to get me out of relapses is worth remembering. Often these were extended efforts, not always immediate or even fast. For instance, upon leaving Aloha House No. 1, she was on mainland and I was out of hotel money so she let me stay in her newly purchased two-bedroom condo in Kihei for a few days. I lied and said I was sober, and it ended up a total disaster. She kicked me out when she returned and needed a place to stay herself, and within days she filed a temporary restraining order (TRO) against me. Right then, I had no home to return to, both on Maui as well as in Long Beach since I lived with her there and the court order transferred.

I stumbled around on the streets for a spell. Karen finally found me maybe a week before Christmas and let me stay. One morning, she drove me to court to address my arrest for the TRO violation, but upon arriving I discovered we were a day early. I screwed up and was frustrated, so leaving the courthouse I had her stop at the mini-mart next door saying I needed tobacco. In reality, I wanted a beer. I bought a 40-ounce cold beer, got back in her car, and cracked it open to sip on the ride. It was probably around 9 a.m. She demanded that I get out, that she wouldn't drive with an open container. I refused, she yelled, some cops just happened to be parked not far away and heard the commotion. They visited, and arrested me for violating the TRO. Again.

I did 10 days in jail, the longest slammer stay ever. I learned, this state does not mess around with restraining order violations. One cellmate said he did a full year on Big Island, for a fourth TRO violation in a 12-month span. The basic rule was, two days jail for first offense, then 10 days, then six months, and a year in jail for the fourth offense. It was standard. Who knew?

After that, Karen took me in temporarily for the rest of the year, but she had to use a free flight ticket by Dec. 31, the end of brutal 2020. So my choice was, return to Long Beach and still live under a TRO which meant not staying in Karen's condo; or staying on island and working through probation terms. I chose the island even without Karen around, and skipping the hassle of transferring probation to L.A. County. It was a big gamble; even the judge, bailiff, and police officer who drove me back to my cell were very surprised. Karen helped me set up places to hide some belongings, like under the cover of one of her cars, plus provided codes to pools at her condos to swim and shower. Finally, she flew off. She had been on island for seven months even though her primary residence was in Long Beach.

I was homeless, and on probation with a judge's order of no alcohol or drugs, and after the 10 days in jail I took that seriously. I'd find nooks to sleep at pandemic-closed government properties, or wherever. I'd use both of Karen's condo pools to charge the phone and shower. I don't know where these survival skills developed, since I wasn't a Boy Scout or big camper previously, but I always seemed to figure it out. Human instinct can be amazing.

Somehow within a few days I met a lady a little older out at the pool of the big condo in central Kihei. She was a sweetheart, a transplant from Missouri who bought a condo there and kind of had her hands full financially. She was working demanding hours at a restaurant at a high-end Wailea resort, and managing. She was tall and slender with darker reddish hair, and super nice. She had an extra room, but was tentative to rent out because she feared the state's big fines for allowing short-term lodging in long-term zoning. But Pacific Shores allowed short-term, otherwise Karen would not have purchased there. I never figured this out, but my friend never said what she expected in rent. She said the room had been rented previously for $1,000 a month, so I did the math and began paying her via an app $33 a night. Not bad at all on this island of exorbitant hotel bed costs.

She was pretty conservative, not in a political sense but in terms of watching out for herself. It was admirable and I respected it. She wouldn't let me stay there while she was away at work. So on those days at 6 a.m. I exited with her, off on my way to find WiFi somewhere to engage my laptop to write for cash. At least I had a nice room with its own shower in a killer location. Things seemed to be improving, and it allowed me to focus on my probation requirements.

My probation officer wound up being a godsend, really a counselor more than a court-appointed rules enforcer. It was only mid-January, and she said my biggest priority at the moment was housing. Probation folks don't like probationers lacking an address. She connected me with a sober living program that ended up playing a huge role in my eventual recovery efforts all the way through this writing. It wasn't immediate, and we had our periodic trials during relapses, but Counseling Alternatives for Recovery Maintenance (CARM) is solid. During my first stint there, I stayed sober nine months. It allowed the opportunity to relax a bit without the anxiety of housing, and adjust to life on my new home island.

* * *

I relapsed in September 2021 and wound up back for **Aloha House No. 2**. This time, with resentment of my previous counselor fresh, and now with a brand-new counselor, my brain thought it was a good idea to do well no matter what, at least in part to spite the first counselor. Yeah, I have mental illness issues. Even after years of Rehab All-Star and AA training, I foolishly held resentments.

The second stay there was a little easier, mainly because I had post-treatment housing set up quickly. My new counselor knew the founder and chief counselor of CARM, and early on arranged a call. I remember how Shelbi of CARM without hesitation said *of course* they'd take me back after the treatment. I felt for my new counselor who was overwhelmed, especially with the computer-entry bureaucracy involved, and wanted to help her and provide a success story to bank on. I never told her this of course but that's how I felt.

I stayed and this time took the coin at the end for completing 42 days. From there, I would be clean and sober for almost two years, all while engaged with the Kaiser Permanente behavioral health program, supported by CARM living, with little to no 12-step involvement. I had this resentment against AA. I felt it would be insane to go back to something that failed me so many times before. In my sick mind, staying sober was a way to stick it to AA.

In the end, the addict beast stuck it to me. House-sitting Karen's new place at the end of July 2023, on an approved pass of several days from CARM allowed due to my longevity there, I discovered a huge bottle of vodka chilling at the bottom of her freezer. I looked past it a few days, but should have trusted my instinct to pour it out. What it tells me is, deep in my mind, I knew eventually I'd tap the bottle, at least a little (haha, right). Everything was lined up to allow it. Days away from the sober living program and its pee tests, no one around to nag, no work obligation … Perfect. I dabbled with sips here and there, into August. By Aug. 8, a historic day with the horrific Maui wildfires all around, personal disaster struck.

Later I learned one of the fires burned right up to the back yards of the homes at the end of our cul-de-sac, no more than maybe 500 feet away. The winds were vicious. I could have been burned to death without waking. I spent the next morning sighing and shaking my head at the close call. Then I saw images of the destruction of Lahaina way up the west coast, where I'd been many times including on first dates, a place I admired for the memories and all the history. That fire was absolutely devastating for anyone living on Maui. That day I packed to finally head home, and not far down the hill I could hear helicopters to the east. Passing by, a neighbor said the fire was still alive, but pushed southeast and around us by stubborn winds. It's just that the firefighters had protected the homes overnight, and the fire veered left. Kihei still wasn't out of the woods. But the damages and lives lost in Lahaina were unimaginable.

I would stay in relapse for months, getting kicked out of CARM again in September but continuing with vodka. Karen hosted me in October, for reasons unknown because I was out of my mind. I decided to head to Los Angeles to help care for my ailing father, who was failing in health and struggling to care for a home by himself with renters he needed to make a mortgage. That was mid-November 2023. After a whirlwind few weeks that included an assault on myself with theft of my phone in Long Beach; three stays in psyche wards; and two weeks in a homeless shelter way up north in Palmdale, I somehow weaseled onto a free Metrolink commuter train ride back to society. While on the train I got help from a good friend dating back to college. I texted asking for a couch for the night in her place in North Hollywood, a stopover en route to Long Beach. She responded, screw a couch, she would get me home. She secured a hotel room near Burbank Airport, and purchased a flight to Maui. It was yet another miracle, by a friend I had become close with once we discovered we both were in recovery. It was early February, 2024.

* * *

With help from a brief stay with Karen, I somehow got back on my feet and into the same sober living house bed at CARM in Kahului not far from the airport. After only about 60 days there, I decided to "adult up" and rent a regular room from a friend in the adjacent community of Wailuku. I was leaving the safety of structure and random pee tests, so I re-enrolled in the intensive outpatient program, and reconnected with my psychiatrist who added yet another med. It was all flowing along swimmingly, then it wasn't. My father passed away in April, shortly after our last contact, a mobile phone video connect on his 80th birthday, April 2. Afterward, I did not drink, but for anxiety I experimented with micro-dosed psilocybin mushrooms, and also with kava and kratom tea. Then I made a final poor choice to create the perfect storm that would send me to my final (so I thought) rehab: a late decision to attend the 40th reunion of my high school class back in Simi Valley. Karen didn't even bother with it, she was too busy. Five brain-fogged days in L.A., followed by five of the same on Maui, and I was back for **Aloha House No. 3** at the end of June 2024.

* * *

There, one Rehab All-Star was actually a five-time Aloha House client. Five times at the same rehab! (Little did I know I'd ultimately do four stays there). That dude was a talkative character, and I hope he gets that general education diploma and finishes drug court once and for all. After he coined out, I discovered another Rehab All-Star – my roommate Glen, a full-on legend in the recovery realm. Addicts will run across someone who was *just worse*, meaning did some crazy-ass shit beyond your own comprehension. It can create a false sense of relief, that *maybe I'm not all that sick*, because *that guy is way sicker!*

Glen had PTSD from serving the Navy and being called to put out oil rig fires during the first Gulf War. He had wild stories both from using and clean time, from around the world. He once met up with the band Aerosmith, their wives, and road crews as they searched for an AA meeting in Japan. They hosted Glen for a big dinner before they all walked off to that night's concert. Glen says he no longer can visit that country, or Australia, due to breaking weird laws or pissing someone off. There is much more legend to tell, but this guy was four years younger than I, had served 15 years in prison, and was displaced by the Maui fire disaster of August 2023 which destroyed the shelter he called home.

Somehow, during the two years I was away, Aloha House management made the operation *even better*. Much of it was due to a more relaxed enforcement of rules, and the erasure of rude or obnoxious program assistants. It was as if a thin foggy layer of anxiety was gone. Sure, clients still did sketchy shit and were punished. For instance, during AH Stay No. 3, a middle-aged guy was caught having a friend hide a log of chewing tobacco cans, not allowed since 2021, near an outdoor trash bin for the client to retrieve. Another dude during a weekly visit to Walmart pre-arranged to meet with a woman, and once caught, the entire trip was canceled on the spot. Everyone suffered due to one person's boneheadedness. It sounded like TTC. The change in 2024 was not having to hear "I'll write you up!" threats all the time, or confusion about rules that sometimes clouded the experience since some PAs either didn't know rules or just made them up.

In short, the Aloha House was like a Bizarro World Salvation Army, a universe where everything is opposite. At Aloha House, they killed you with kindness, and the graduation rates reflected it. The number of clients who left or were kicked out before getting their coin was very low; definitely opposite of the "tough love" facilities I survived.

After being away so long, and a bit more developed in my recovery, I noticed little things previously overlooked. One of them, and maybe this is just an age thing, is all the chattering. Idle chat among clients, like before and even *during* group sessions, was distracting and annoying. There was chatter at night in dorms, while you tried to relax or read. The talking was incessant. New rehabbers should know: have patience, avoid resentments, and maintain focus on what's important, namely the lessons and your program. It's easy to dislike some colleagues around you, who also are going through a difficult life period. Maintain empathy, and laugh off minor disturbances.

Much of this has to do with what we in recovery call "war stories," tales from using or drinking. It seems everyone wants to *out-do* each other. You'll hear every crazy story, like the time Glen was upset with a dude in jail so he stole the guy's toothbrush, stuck it way up his butthole, then returned it to a sink for his antagonist to discover. Legend! There will be more than one Jail All-Star, and when two or more JAS's get together, they will talk at length about POs (probation officers), ACOs (assistant correction officers who patrol jails), eating meals quickly, cheap rubber slippers, parole, probation, UAs, drug court, and more. Jail talk is constant. These guys all seem to remember each other, too. I only did 10 days in the slammer here, but afterward ran into two dudes "on the outside." Guys in Aloha House got excited when newcomers entered detox; they seemed to wait for each new guy because they might know them from the streets or jail.

Young guys will talk nonstop about the mundane, like video games, comic book action movies, or anime, etc. Like the girls they know, friends they might share, judges, probation officers, bitching about parents, whatever. Topics veer all over the place and it's constant. It's as if they just re-discovered their voice and worked the voice box back into shape.

Some new guys in group sessions will try to *eat the elephant with one bite* – a term first directed at me by the guy at the Sally who stabbed the other guy. That is, you arrive new to a program, maybe fresh out of a relapse, with limited knowledge about getting well, yet immediately share in meetings. This usually doesn't last long, until someone says or hints to shut up and listen. These fresh talkative folks can be called "instant counselors," or "counselors in training." I did it upon my first in-house AA meeting at the Sally, for which the stabber more than once chided me for "trying to eat the elephant with one bite!" It took a while to figure out what he meant.

Repeating the point above, some colleagues in rehab you will dislike. Unfortunately, unlike in the real world where you can walk away or purposely avoid annoyances, in rehab *you're stuck with them*, often in close quarters. It might very well be a roommate. They might talk too much, or seem to pick on you, or just rub you the wrong way. New rehabbers should expect this, and get past it, quickly. Fighting or making threats will get you ejected. I found myself self-talking in such instances: "It isn't worth it, Keith. Let it be." Or, "Laugh it off!" Sometimes I borrowed from AA and tried to kill them with kindness, or prayed for them. In the end, most troublemakers get themselves kicked out; even roommates don't last forever. Things pass and the entire experience is not permanent or even long-term. Deal with it.

Remember the main goal: to get clean and sober and stay that way. Rehab situations are temporary. Time in a rehab is miniscule compared to a lifetime. A blink of an eye, really. Don't let personalities bump you off your recovery track. I let that guy in my first sober living house on Maui bother me for no real reason, Pasty Man who I later saw talking to himself in a beach parking lot. In rehabs and recovery situations, people with serious mental ailments abound.

I let a life loser get in my grill, letting a resentment brew. It mixed with other resentments I failed to identify and address, and created one of those perfect storms for relapse. Very often, relapses are not the result of a single event, situation, or feeling. Many times it's a *combination* of things aggravating your brain's neural pathways simultaneously. It's a reason they recommend daily doses of AA at the beginning. I can vouch that I need at least an hour every day reminding myself that I have a mental malady. Whether that means attending a 12-step meeting, or talking with others in recovery, or doing anything related to the recovery effort, I need to do something daily. It serves to remind you that you are sick; and treating that illness outweighs in importance any perceived slight. There's an AA slogan all members eventually come across: *Live and let live.*

New rehabbers will be tested, maybe from a 12-step program, by other people, or even from a spirit. What you train for in recovery is the *ability to pass these tests.* The AA book is not all about alcohol. In fact, the word *alcohol* surfaces only in the first 60 or so pages of the main book. After that, the thrust is to establish a healthy and spiritual way of living, one so fulfilling and serene that there is no urge or need to drink or use substances. The AA big book is a user's manual to guide humans to learn how to live better. It's about *learning how to respond to life*. Personalities within the program can (and will) irritate, something which as mentioned must be overcome. As they say in AA literature and meetings, "Principles before personalities."

In rehab, you'll have to live with and accept a whole lot of differing personalities. You *will* get annoyed. You learn much about the importance of patience. I remember something Dad once said, about lacking empathy. Somewhere in AA's big book it says that when confronted with a troublesome person, *pray for them*. Remember that the other person, like you, is not well. There is a lot about avoiding resentments in that book, for good reason.

Also helpful is something counselors have said more than once. Remember that the colleagues around you are also alcoholics or addicts going through a difficult time personally and emotionally. You don't know about their thoughts and emotions, whether one wrong word could set them off to pack and leave. And leaving could be a death sentence.

Try to show empathy for all, love your brothers and sisters (but not too much), listen to your counselors, PAs, and in group, and put your recovery before anything else, like my old Redgate counselor said.

* * *

I heard it while in **Aloha House No. 3** within the first weeks. While I was familiar with most of the lessons, it was helpful to have "refresher" sessions, to cement messages into my thinking, and constantly remind myself that I have a life-threatening illness. I cannot emphasize enough this last part: Addicts can easily forget we are in fact very ill, and then try things normal people handle routinely, but we simply *cannot*. Something I should have gotten daily in meetings, or through talking with all the sober people among my All-Star Support Group. Maintenance help is rarely far away when you leave rehab. There are AA or NA meetings open at all times. Those you can't reach physically, you can do now via livestream apps like Zoom, thanks to skills perfected during the pandemic lockdown.

During what I thought was the last Aloha House stay, when halfway done in late July 2024, I figured out where I failed at 130 days sober. My father passed in April, and it was not a surprise as his health had been failing for some time. I was actually relieved for him. He was ready to reconnect with Mom in Heaven.

However I repeated the mistake made when Mom passed in 2016: I didn't change my routine, and did not seek assistance with the grieving process. Both times I chose to keep doing daily what I did prior to the death. I needed *more* meetings, whether in AA, or via my behavioral health program or with close friends, not fewer. So entering May, it was as if I was traversing a big ice sheet, that was cracking badly with each step. I should have reached out to numerous people. By this time I had so many friends familiar with my recovery that there was no excuse to not tap into one or two or eight of them. They are always available, and most willing to help.

In May, even though I have doctor-prescribed meds for anxiety, I chose to experiment with micro-dosing magic mushrooms, and legal beverages like kava and kratom. As my favorite punk rocker once sang, "I was almost over, my time was nearly gone. But in a sudden rush I could almost touch the things that I'd done wrong." That's how I felt toward the end of Aloha House No. 3. I no longer act like this well-experienced recovery expert. I was much less talkative in the last rehabs. I followed the advice of a long-past sponsor: "Share only if you believe what you say might help another person." I tried only to supplement what group hosts were trying to impress, based on real-life experiences. I don't speak up in groups just to hear my own voice, like counselors-in-training.

I look back on all the other rehab stays with awe. How did I survive 15 months over a 21-month period at the Sally? Three or four months in TTC or Redgate? It doesn't seem real, compared against the weeks of programs on Maui. Of the 149 months from my first rehab stay in March 2012 to July 2024, I'd spent *22% of my life in rehabs*. Almost a quarter of the time I was alive during that period, I was in inpatient treatment. Tack onto that about three years in sober living houses, mostly in CARM on Maui, and time in shelters, and I'm confident to say I spent 40% of my time over a dozen years confined to something that forbade alcohol or drugs. About six years of my life in total lost to institutional care.

When I began this writing, I was 58, but in reality I'd lived about 52 years. Add years lost to bat-shit crazy addiction, and you get about a decade's worth of nothingness. I'd lost my wife, kids, house, car, friends and family members, freedom, reputation, my community, and more. In short, all that mattered. What I thought was the last rehab may have come as a shocker, after 23 months sober, but it ended up being a nice refresher course, a time to reflect and honestly assess myself and life. What can I do further to prevent this?

I know it is very serious. Now, the blackouts started too quickly, the severity worsened, the pain overwhelmed. There is a strong likelihood that I *won't have another recovery in me*, as old-timers say. I was already lucky to have as many as I did. To newcomers: **get it right the first time**, and avoid the Russian roulette of relapse.

* * *

Much of that resurfaced in the 2024 rehab. I'd encounter clients being honest saying they were there only because of parole or probation. Sometimes younger clients have a hard time admitting or realizing just how *big* their problem is. It's enormous, if you land in *just one rehab*. If you get into rehab, you have a serious problem with alcohol or drugs. I remember in an AA meeting long ago, a fellow alcoholic said something to the effect of, if you ever had *one* problem because of alcohol, you're an alcoholic. Anything: a fight, scuffle, fall, arrest, vandalism, violence, etc., and you're an alcoholic. It reminded me of my earliest alcohol-driven escapades.

In the middle of my senior year of high school, one night at a friend's mini house party, I realized I was drunk and needed sleep. I lived in the same housing tract, but still only made it about three blocks driving my car before pulling over, and parking in front of a random house in the dark. I jumped into the back seat and fell asleep. Eventually a police officer knocked on my window. The neighbor in the house I parked in front of reported suspicious activity. To the officers, my eyes appeared jumpy, and they took me to the station. I learned later they had suspicion of use of PCP, known as angel dust, an exotic drug (which eventually I'd try once, determining it is the worst drug experience possible).

Dad and my uncle Bob were called away from a night of card playing and socializing with the wives, which had to be nerve-racking since I'm sure they drank beer. That's what the Jajko brothers did. The cops inspected my arms closely, for the veins, looking for a syringe spot. They focused on a tiny mole on the inside of my left wrist, which is still there, still looking like a tiny needle poke. But I had never injected drugs (nor ever would by myself; someone else did for me a third of a century later). Ultimately they asked several times to think hard about where I'd been and what I might have ingested. I finally remembered smoking a clove cigarette at the party, and said so. Amazingly they said yes, they had heard that clove cigarettes could make your eyes jittery. Wow. They released me to Dad.

It was a close call, which just seemed fortunate. I lucked out, oh well. Dad warned to be more careful out there, but everyone agreed it was wise to pull over instead of drunken driving. It wasn't until years later when the guy in AA said that *any* problem caused by alcohol meant alcoholism. Then I thought about it and remembered being caught the very first time I drank away from my parents, a couple of beers while walking with buddies to a junior high dance. We were grabbed by the vice principal hanging out next to the physical education locker rooms, before the dance opened. At that moment, the guy who'd given me the beer ran down a big slope into dark athletic fields to escape, in response to a vice principal yelling at us. Me and another friend froze, busted, watching Akrop hop over the ledge and down the hill into darkness. It was ugly in the administration office, and at home.

I had no idea this was a premonition of things to come. In the interrogation waiting for my parents to retrieve me, I called the vice principal a dick, fairly loudly, complicating everything. (It did make me a semi-legend on campus, though). Basically, I realized that I was an alcoholic for a very long time.

All this would return in memories in later rehabs. It takes about a week in detox to regain my balance and ability to speak in complete sentences; then 14 to 16 days for the brain to feel normal and fully functional. Thereafter, the brain seems to recover quickly. By the third week, shit not remembered in eons seemed to pop up, prompted by a reading or something said. It happens a lot in group and 12-step meetings, when people say something that seems eerily familiar.

At Aloha House No. 3, I did more Bible reading than usual, not necessarily by choice but because Bible study was available every morning in the men's smoking section. I also read a book that snuck God into the plot consistently. It helped much to slow down, breathe, relax, let things pass, and appreciate the moment and day to come. Little things that could set me off each day are more easily managed with a relaxed mind.

It's a huge lesson for new rehabbers, one which doesn't require Scriptures: remain calm. Things pass. If possible, avoid drama or situations you *know* will impact your mood. Pause when agitated. *Play the tape forward.* Imagine if you made a certain choice, like losing your temper, and how the dominoes would fall. Play out scene after scene in your head. I yell at Brian, he yells back, I slap him, get ejected, maybe go to jail, perhaps end up back on the streets. If the tape ends badly like that – injury, jail, death, homelessness, etc. – move on. I kind of like repeating something from the Monty Python movie with King Arthur: *run away!*

Annoyances are exacerbated by the limitations of space. Some facilities are not large, or are always crowded, with a wide range of ages and personalities. I was in my late 40s at my first rehab. By that age, teenage-level behavior by people in their 20s or even 30s is not easily tolerated. You want to bark out at dudes. If a particular habit by an individual annoys you, it probably will get repeated. You can spend a lot of time in groups daydreaming about how you would beat the fuck out of someone.

This is key in recovery: much is about improving your *odds for success*. Recovery is hard. It helps to do things to improve your chances. Like quitting tobacco, or attending 12-step meetings consistently. It's likely that someone or something will influence you to act in ways that could *decrease* the odds for success. Don't surrender that power over yourself to another person, or even institution (like a rehab program or 12-step program, things I held resentments against). That's all channel noise distorting important messages you need to absorb and apply.

In the latter part of the 2024 rehab, I got pretty good at managing this. I do imagine, however, how difficult it would be without prior experience. Rehabs don't always do this purposely, but they are full of tests. Annoying people, silly rules, sillier consequences, rude or unprofessional support staff … some which have contributed to knocking me out. Not got me kicked out, necessarily, though that did happen twice. But incidents or situations messed up my thinking. I walked out of rehabs before completing program, which is a waste of time.

If the goal is long-term sobriety or clean time, focus is imperative. Keep an open mind, about things like a power greater than yourself, or even God, or meditation and mindfulness. Accepting your illness, and what it does to you, and what it will take to manage, is crucial. A willingness to change almost everything in your life helps. Fear of change wipes out a lot of addicts. It's a reason for the *one day at a time* mantra. Addicts can't afford to think too far into the future, because doing so has no end. If you start thinking about next week, soon you'll be imagining the calendar and dates and other challenges approaching in coming weeks or months. It fuels anxiety, which in the end can kill. My attitude when doing well is this. If I can get between the sheets of my bed at night at the end of the day clean and sober, I won. I *won the chance to try again the next day*. I try not to think much beyond the current day and maybe the day immediately following. Never further than that.

* * *

A funny story from AH No. 3. For this round, the program began importing clients from other islands which might not have rehab options, like Big Island. (A year later, clients from Molokai began arriving). During stay No. 3, there was a guy named Jessie G. who kind of took me in at the beginning and was very helpful. He always told stories about fights with his girlfriend, like the time she busted his car windshield. I guess they had a habit of playing "Tag, You're It!" with each other's car windows. So, being a smart addict, he once took off his rear window and duct-taped it to the front, "to abide by the law." To which I asked, *Which is?* He said, "Duct tape to stop leaks when it rains. It leaks eventually, though." Another time he and the gal smashed *all* the windows of each other's cars. Once they made up, he realized, *what do we do now?* So he drove around with no windows, kids in the back seat and all. Cops would pull him over and laugh. I asked, is that legal? "Yes. Everyone in the car just has to be wearing glasses."

You learn a lot in rehabs.

* * *

For insight into what to expect during a typical week in rehab, following is a detailed journal of everything that happened for a full week during what I thought was my Final Tour Rehab.

NEAR THE END OF THE 2024 REHAB, OR ALOHA HOUSE NO. 3

Prologue

After six days in detox, I was walked over to residential – 38 beds for men and women. It had been three years, but the layout was unchanged. Same dorms, dining deck, classroom, main office, dirt volleyball court. Some staff remained but new personnel arrived. Something noticeable was that, somehow, they made the place even better. I noticed PAs were less stressed and more forgiving, and that a few weasel staffers were gone. Then I noticed a new director of the entire program, and knew someone cleaned house. Gone were PAs who harassed and constantly threatened write-ups. Sure, periodically we'd get lectured as a group about certain rules or situations, but overall they treated us as adults, and we reacted well. It was refreshing.

It resulted in less drama, allowing more energy to focus in group. Plus, there is a lot of physical exercise time built into the Aloha House schedule. I sucked at volleyball at first, but as a former beach player, I knew to just keep playing. I improved as my balance and hand-eye coordination returned. I was the oldest fahka out there. We also did a beach visit every Friday morning, and of course kickball every Monday afternoon with my old counselor who was competitive as hell which kept it entertaining and fun. I didn't always play kickball for fear of injury. Sure enough, the very first kick my last game, I pulled a quad muscle in my right leg. I still legged out a single. I can say my final kick-ball at-bat resulted in a safe hit. (Years prior in the very last soccer game of my life, while at Redgate, I scored two goals including an incredible planned play where I deflected a corner kick with an old side-kick maneuver learned from old-school hacky-sack. My buddy Nolan executed the corner kick perfectly and says he still remembers the play. The goalie didn't even move. It was hilarious.)

Most often on Monday afternoons I would walk, circling the huge grass areas of the park where kickball was played on a single diamond in a corner.

I'd pepper in push-ups, leg lifts, and stretches. After cutting back on meal consumption after a week of gorging, I exercised and started losing weight. I began to appreciate looking better.

Early on, I determined this was my Rehab Farewell Tour. I'd just done three years without a rehab, a record during a 12-year period of trying. I was now old, which makes relapses as embarrassing as they are painful. I realized what had gone wrong; and knew what I needed to do to not replay that tape. I needed to engage with sober people every day, with no days off from recovery. I needed to actively work to keep my sobriety, including getting re-engaged with AA if that's what it would take.

I planned to move out of the private room I'd rented a few months in Wailuku, to a town that had more AA meetings and options. I would get away from the old central Maui suburbs where I'd lived over three years, to a town with beaches from top to bottom. I would make beach days a big part of my program. In Kihei, they have AA meetings on grasses right at the shoreline.

With that decided – and a young, energetic, and caring counselor helped – I could have been done in a couple of weeks. But my insurance gave me 45 days, and since I always tell others to take as many days as they'll allow, I had to complete this whole stay. No way could I leave early. How would I explain trouble if it developed? I couldn't.

It's important to note that by this point I no longer had to work. I was not in a relationship, nor had any real commitments. I sympathize with young rehabbers who have to handle all this rehab boringness while worried about keeping a job, paying bills, keeping the partner, having a roof over your head at night, and more. I dealt with some of that early on in rehabs, but by the end these issues were gone.

This allowed a rare situation. For the first time, I could relax and really digest everything before me. I had this conversation with an Aloha House staffer named Herman one day. We know it's hard to focus on recovery when you have no home. Or have no money or a job. These matters are almost impossible to keep out of your thoughts. While in rehab, there is plenty of down time at night before sleep to reflect, or let the mind go wild. Even during groups, I daydream. If any stresses are present at any moment, they can dominate thoughts (and worries). It takes a superstar to keep your mind on topic during the hours and hours in groups. God help those with housing, money, health, or relationship woes.

During this "final" rehab, somewhere around mid-point, the clientele turned over. I was around a different group of colleagues each half. Most who were there in July with me coined out to graduate. The second half, the crew seemed to have fewer jail veterans and drug court students. There seemed to be more newbies than usual, a lot of them young or at least not quite adults. Seriously, one day a colleague and I had a discussion, where he said he'd never seen a group in rehab that immature. I just laugh and ride it out. It does, however, make me wonder if I can last another two weeks.

Tonight, as with every Wednesday, there's an optional off-campus 12-step meeting they van us to attend. This night, like most others, I passed. I get tired after full days of group, and additionally, I dislike night meetings. Going off campus, we wouldn't arrive back until 9 p.m. at earliest. On this night, I wrote at that moment, it was just two wake-ups before beach time Friday, then another weekend of nothingness.

* * *

Josh of AIA in Lake Arrowhead, during our second stay together once randomly asked, "Is it just me, or are there a bunch of dildos here?" It's interesting how the overall group can be much different just days apart. I realized at that moment in Aloha House, finishing July 2024, we seemed to have too many dildos around. I looked forward to many coin-outs. Then again, after that, I'd get just a short period of peace before I too was coined out. And, who knows what fucking new guys (FNGs) would arrive by then?

While I still had rehab fatigue, there were at least moments of good laughs remaining. Big Brian of Big Island one morning was pissed because getting meds was postponed until after breakfast. He made a big stink about it, in the thick pidgin language style of true locals. Then later that morning, in med line I accidentally skipped past him to get meds before his daily blood pressure screen. "Asshole Keith," he mumbled with a sly smile. Haha!

Around that time, I started what I hoped would be my last rehab practical joke. This old-time AA dude in the other dorm complained often about roosters that would crow close to his window early mornings at ungodly hours. For a few days his complaints stalled for whatever reason, which is probably what triggered my idea. It was funny hearing him whine every morning while arriving (usually late) to the first group. What if someone did something to attract chickens near that corner of his dorm? How might we force the matter, and trigger him to keep complaining about roosters every day? My thoughts probably came from my father, who seemed to relish in prolonging someone's misery with what he thought was something really funny.

So at that Sunday's store run, the Ted Jajko in me came out. I bought a lot of small boxes of cheap raisins and some sunflower seeds. Back at the rehab I picked my moment and tip-toed around to the rear of Dorm A to toss a lot of raisins right outside Whiner's window, and a small cupful of seeds. However, a client who lives in that same dorm saw me leave from the side of the structure after raisin drop No. 1. I approached him and explained that it was just a joke, and why. Days later, my roommate Thomas said that Whiner asked him for "insight" into me. Something like, "I heard Keith's dumping raisins near my room. I'm trying to figure out how to get him back." Not exactly subtle.

Situations like that are somewhat concerning, since not everyone in recovery has a sense of humor. Anyway, I had plenty of peanuts and seeds to drop for weeks, and money to get more. But in the end, it wound up being the greatest practical joke backfire ever. You see, Whiner worked in the kitchen, which happened to be upstairs pretty much adjacent to my dorm, in which my room was closest. The window was maybe two feet from my head in bed. For a couple of weeks I would walk outside and find remnants of meals peppered around the grass in front of my window. One morning, I noticed a shitload of *chickens feasting on these large items, which upon closer inspection turned out to be ... tamales. Full, cooked tamales. Well played, Whiner, well played.*

One other memory was not a practical joke, but something I did to help reduce noise near my room and it kept me giggling for weeks. My room was next to the south door of our building, which faced the side of the kitchen. Outside that door is a little concrete landing pad, connected to a short concrete trail to the main road that leads to the kitchen and office. We didn't have a big wooden deck to sit and relax like Dorm A. Boomhauer one day found a metal chair and decided to set it on the landing, to sit and shoot the breeze with anyone who walked by. And Boomhauer talked a lot, even though I couldn't understand most of his pidgin. He mumbled too fast. After a few days of having my reading disrupted by concrete pad discussions, I'd had enough, and discretely took the chair and moved it to the other side of the building, near the north door. Well, Boomhauer found it immediately and later that day there it was, near my room again.

So it was my move. Once the area was deserted, I took the chair and very carefully walked it all the way around the building up the parking lot and around the kitchen, and left it on a big faux wood smoking deck far from my room. Then the fun began. Boomhauer went nuts. "Someone took my chair!" he would say over and over to anyone nearby. Actually he said a lot more but few understood. We just knew it was about some chair. I knew exactly which chair, and where it was located. It took a while, but eventually he saw the chair ... because he smoked on the deck. Why it took so long for him to identify it made the whole incident even funnier. He returned it to the concrete pad, but soon after without prompt a staffer took it and hid it for good, reason unknown. Fuckin' Boomhauer of Big Island. At least Brian I could understand.

At AH Nos. 3 and 4, I befriended a true Rehab All-Star who went by the name Spencer, who then had been with me at Aloha House three times. He was my last roommate during my first stay, and we always seemed to run into each other at the main bus depot during periods where we both were sober or in sober living houses. Godspeed, Craig! Hope to not see you in rehab yet again!

* * *

In the Personal Journey group one morning, a discussion developed regarding how drugs hurt us physically, yet we still went ahead and ingested. One client said, "I can memorize and recite all this shit all I want, but it won't stop me (from using)." Reminds me of how many times I had heard the lectures about physical damage from alcohol, yet there I was, because of ingesting too much alcohol. My colleague was right. Us serious addicts didn't care about our health. The substance was more important.

The days remaining began to dwindle, and I realized that many clients who helped get me get this far in this rehab were long gone. I heard from the current fellas who went to outside meetings, that they'd seen old colleagues like "Black Keith," and that they were doing well and obviously attending meetings. Near this end stage, only two "old-timers" remained: a guy who loaded me with instant coffee on Day 1 so I was forever in debt; and Breezy, a female I befriended when she went to court and we did not expect her back. While she sat in a staff car awaiting the ride to court (and possibly jail), I ran up, tapped the window, and when she looked I thumped my chest hard and said aloud, "Keep the faith!" Later that day when she returned to walk into the middle of a group session, she got a resounding ovation. I was elated, even though in reality she and I had never shared more than a few words. I just felt it was so unfair for someone to be taken out of a rehab where she'd already dedicated weeks, to stick in jail where you get little recovery-related attention. I must say, the justice system on Maui is, ahem, different.

The new crowd was so much different than the original gang. Not as many smokers remained, or even dudes in need of smokes. For a spell, a lot of newcomers came in. It hit me that it happens in every rehab: this mass turnover, where people you thought you'd miss, or felt like you'd connect with on the outside, are forgotten. It's a reminder that a return to the Real World is approaching. It's around this near end point of a person's program where you notice changes *in personalities. Guys who were cocky and clique-prone suddenly become quiet and reserved; or they show signs of being* scared. *Their posture changes, facial expressions become more solemn. Suddenly they realize this coddled camp life is about to end, and shit is about to get real, and fast.*

At that point in The Final Rehab, I wasn't feeling it. It was the first time where my immediate future was known. Housing, what to do, etc. Immediate post-treatment housing causes grief for many modern rehabbers. Money and jobs are up there, but where to live is hard to ignore when you face having nowhere to go.

Post-rehab housing most often involves sober living house programs, or houses that act like sober living environments, which costs money. Clients lean on counselors heavily for help, but these staffers are not required to do so. To the best of my knowledge, they don't provide schooling on this topic on your way to a substance abuse counseling certificate. Many institutions try hard to keep clients in sober living houses they separately operate, or direct clients to an intensive outpatient program. This post-rehab period is known as after care, *and I cannot emphasize enough how vital it is for graduated rehabbers. I didn't have lengthy stints of sobriety, post-rehab, until I tried IOP.*

I know a sober living program on island that almost always has a bed open. I have conveyed this to rehab clients and staff; and also mentioned a church that would cover a first month's rent. The information did not seem to attract much interest. If I was a counselor, I would compile a toolbox of every housing option known. Few at Aloha House seemed interested. Maybe I'm wrong, but I remember some Redgate counselors who took finding housing seriously, one even calling me twice to inquire about beds in the COA men's program. Oh well, I thought, at least I didn't have to live through a Compton nightmare all over again, on Maui.

At the very end of rehab, past the 30-day mark, group sessions get repetitive. Some topics cycle through and get repeated, purposely, for the benefit of newcomers and at the expense of people who'd been there a while. Some groups are based on outdated printouts, which to me is unattractive in an ever-evolving field. Additionally, some group facilitators take it too seriously as if they are college instructors. These hosts think they need to use every last second, and maybe even more, to make some climatic point at the end. At the very end of group sessions, clients are indifferent and impatient. You get tired, and your back or ass hurts from sitting so long on hard chairs. Most group sessions should be shorter and to the point, and the end time respected, in my opinion.

Other facilitators are just dry, going over a workbook or handouts, making us read paragraphs then asking for reactions, questions, etc. This tact can make 90 minutes seem like half a day or more. Eventually, it's hard to return after breaks in the longer 90- or 120-minute meetings. With just a week remaining, it's always tempting. I skipped out once or twice at The Final Rehab. Not a major infraction, and afternoon naps feel good.

***

During the very last week, I felt fully "grouped out," a mindless almost zombie-like state of walking to sessions in a daze and sitting still staring into space for good chunks of time. The repetition can get grueling. But that's what it takes to get these messages to germinate in our beat-up brains. With my post-treatment plans solidified and that typical worry out of the way, I was very bored.

At the end, I realized more details about what ailed me, and maybe why. But ... it was not always explained how this information would keep me sober. I know I'm mentally ill; you don't have to spend much energy proving it. A final guest speaker there may have provided the best advice: be humble, pray, and be grateful.

A WEEK IN THE LIFE AT ALOHA HOUSE, AUGUST 2024

Monday, Aug. 8

Opening. Around 6:50 a.m., Big Island Brian and another client talk loudly right outside my door. The discussion involves showers, as they stand outside that particular bathroom, one of two at either end of our dorm. They are staring at a program schedule posted to a wall just outside my room door. It forced me out of bed and into the hallway. Following is a discussion I found amusing:

BRIAN: "What is Hygiene class?"

ME: "Nap time."

BRIAN: "Yeah. What is *that?*"

ME: "Their reminder that we need to take showers. Some guys don't, and say they don't have the time. By putting it on the schedule, they point to that hour as time you could be showering."

BRIAN: "Some guys afraid of water. We washing the vans, so I shot the hose over the van, to get him wet."

OTHER CLIENT: "I think maybe he has rabies."

BRIAN: "Yeah, people afraid of water, might get rabies."

It is at this moment that I walk away to go ring a bell.

***

In reality, this is how the day began: Eyes open and awake at 5 a.m., but not actually out of bed until **6:05 a.m.**, to make a cup of instant coffee, and get tobacco into my system. (I smoked the first three weeks here; snuck in chewing tobacco for the final weeks). Had a second cup of coffee at 7, and immediately got my morning meds right when they began distributing them. I have to visit the front desk every morning to take three psychiatric medicines. Big Island Brian is in line behind me. He always seems to be in the med line.

7:20 a.m. I stay near a clock so I can go ring my first bell of the day, 10 minutes before the **7:30 a.m.** Morning Meditation session we all sit through to start weekdays.

I meander up exterior stairs up onto the dining deck adjacent to the kitchen, and find a bell and rope attached to a wall a little higher than eye level, and pull to ring the fucker loud two or three times. Then I walk to the classroom for the half-hour wake-up session.

Bell Ringer was my assigned daily chore. I mentioned before, at almost every rehab I assumed some important volunteer role, whether I wanted to or not. Usually it was because of my big mouth and complaining. That's what happened here, on top of the fact that the people who assign chores knew I made it to class every day on time and could be reliable. Bell Ringer is not a fun responsibility, because you have to find clocks and watch them, and go ring the bell multiple times each day, for groups and meals, or occasionally for a special event or request. It was kind of like the Voice of Redgate role I did, only using a bell instead of PA announcements (e.g. "Group B, you have group in 10 minutes," followed by the same announcement broadcast into every hallway and room with five minutes to spare, a la my predecessor Jenn who I dubbed the original Voice of Redgate). At Aloha House I did get to flirt with the girls sitting near the bell. That deck was their smoking section and they sat right under the bell, rarely with any staff nearby. It was a good time to sneak idle chats and random jokes.

In morning meditation, a staffer will speak briefly, then we go around the room and say one thought, one feeling, urges, and something we're grateful for. Two mornings a week, a staffer walked us through a guided meditation – not a bad way to start a day. It's brief, and few are sleepy since big food is next. Almost always, one client will be sad about missing loved ones, or express a feeling of burnout. It comes and goes; you hear it all.

This morning, a cool PA named Herman asked us to talk about the Word (of God); what we have *thought* about doing, compared with what you know protects you. Something like that. It was way early for my brain to fully absorb instructions. He then asked us to re-play our thoughts about what happens *IF* we drink. One clients says, "Every time I drink, I lose something … something important to me. Last time I drank, I lost a good relationship. You always lose something." To which I added, "I call this playing the tape forward." I made a mental note that some PAs speak very well with us, like Herman, especially when it comes to the Word. Herman adds, "Enjoy this feeling, continue to be the best version of yourself. Think about the opportunity God has given you, because some people have to wait months to get into a place like this." Amen, braddah.

When my turn came, I mentioned how we get cared for here, with no rent, good free food … once that ends, then WHAM! The real world, rent, car, insurance, kids, bills, and more. That's where the real change begins. Regarding his own recovery, Herman ends with, "That's why I fight every day. So no one can come in and take my place."

8 a.m. Breakfast. Almost everyone over-eats. Rehab veterans know to skip the rice, and avoid returning for second helpings which are available almost every meal session. My only treat is when they have chocolate-chip or blueberry muffins. I passed on ice cream one night when a PA was nice enough to buy a shitload for us all. I stopped doing sugar in November 2022. Today, breakfast burrito! A massive undertaking.

After, I visited the main office to retrieve a pack of cigarettes I'd stored there inside plastic see-through drawers they kept for clients, to give away to my new roommate. On this stay, I didn't get any cash until two or three weeks in. Once I did (delivered by my angel Karen), I bought a lot of cigarette packs because I'd borrowed so many and wanted to pay folks back. Plus, chew was banned, so I felt forced to smoke. During the same initial store visits for me, after surviving being "dark" for the first two weeks, I was able to secretly buy cans of chew, and slowly wean off the smokes. I didn't mind having all the extra cig packs; I was paying the community back for carrying me for weeks while broke. Don't underestimate how hard the rehab road is for those addicted to tobacco with no money. Try to enter rehab with at least some dough.

Then I had a brief break between groups, which I spent line-editing chapters of a book written by my friend James Swanson ("Super Stoked"), from printed sheets Karen had delivered during a visitation. It takes a while to get settled into rehab, with restrictions early on, but eventually you can enjoy some perks as long as you behave. I did this until it was time to go ring the bell for the start of group sessions for the week. The first was Creative Writing from 9 to 10 a.m.

9 a.m. Creative Writing. Notable for this session is that we had to carry all the chairs from the classroom to arrange the dining deck up the outdoor stairs, for a two-day project to get the classroom an air-conditioning unit. The project was teased to us every time I came here, and finally a cooler classroom was arriving. Adjustments like this happen in rehabs for capital improvement projects, just not all as major as my last stay at the Sally when I was moved from a three-bed room to a barracks of seven. Addicts don't do well with change; big sudden changes can drive some to the brink of insanity. Oh, the questions, constantly. Even after staff provides answers, clients ask again. The same question, repeat. Even if the answer was provided just *moments* prior. It's just how it is. Most people listen and gather information before asking questions. Others ask questions whenever they feel like it, or when their ears start working again. If they feel like it later, they might research.

There also can be jealousy and resentments from other clients, especially if colleagues suspect *special treatment*. I noticed the "I want one, too!" stances fairly often. It was something I hadn't experienced since my public school days. For instance the week prior, per *direction from my counselor* to try something that made me uncomfortable, I was allowed to present a writing tip for this very creative writing group session. It ended up taking the entire time of the class. I wrote instructions about keeping sentences short; then made a brief writing assignment for clients to try it. I found it to be a wonderful, different experience, being on the "other side" presenting to a rehab audience. However, it generated jealousy or mild resentment from certain clients, as if I was given *special treatment*. It didn't matter that I was asked to do this by my own counselor, so this group host let me do it last-minute. She was not pre-warned; I asked her as she sat before the group before start time. Anyone else could ask to do something like that, if they wished. The jealousy thing reared its head later on.

During this creative writing session, the counselor prompted us with, "What is your dream life, and the steps needed to get there?" This session is usually easy, because everyone stays quiet for an extended period while we get to listen to soft island reggae. Then, we get to volunteer to read what we wrote, and kill the rest of the hour. There was some debate about speaking up so everyone could hear, especially with all the cackling chickens, er, young talkative clients. Somehow we managed to finish, and got to the all-important break. There, a Pavlovian conditioning seems evident at the scheduled group end time (though without bells; those are only for *start times*). Once dismissed, there's a stampede to the smoking areas or back to dorms, laundry room, or phone.

10:15 a.m. Group No. 2 on the day. My own counselor hosted this group, one of three each week when we go over, word for word, text from the My Personal Journal workbook. We again did this on the dining deck outdoors. Outside groups are different. At least you get fresh air and different sounds and smells. Watching clouds while hearing birds chirp is better than staring at white walls or a dry-erase board. My counselor this day was pinch-hitting for an absent counselor who usually hosted. This allows no time for her to prepare, and it's arguably the most boring topic each week. My Personal Journey is a school-like workbook published in 2014 – a decade prior! We read word for word, page for page, giving time for everyone to write and fill in various blanks, and then an opportunity to share if desired. It's a super boring book, outdated, with a lot of "*No shit?*" sections, such as losing stuff to substance abuse; alcohol's effects; mass details about various drugs;

a lot of pages detailing AA's early steps; and time and money management. (Note: Aloha House dumped use of this workbook by 2025).

The difference here compared with other rehabs is the people sharing. Just when you think you've seen every personality type, you get introduced to new ones. I still can't define my first roommate during the Final Rehab. Glen was the Gulf War veteran with PTSD and a gnarly addiction to drugs. Here, we also get to hear the backgrounds of local islanders, see guys covered in tattoos, including on their face and neck, or women with horrific tales of abuse. Some stubborn personalities leave program early. Others, mostly old-timers, speak at length about what's bothering them that day or moment, things like not being able to see their kids grow, or riding a motorcycle.

It's only late morning and already I'm super sleepy, and semi-bored, but experienced enough to tap tools learned over the years. I instinctively know when to actively *eat the clock*. It's a key skill, I've found. Time seems to move faster when you do things while sitting in group, like making to-do lists, writing out post-program plans, composing a book, etc., while still kind of listening to the facilitator and your colleagues. I'm Pro+ Level at this.

My counselor lets us out barely a few minutes short of the 11:45 a.m. end time, and I take a brief nap before ringing the bell for lunch. Today it's split-pea soup, salad, cheesy bread, green beans, and tea. Not fancy, but all tasty. Afterward, I did my post-meals chore. I swept the stairs up to the dining deck, and checked the trash can up there. Then it was back to my room, which happened to be the closest to the kitchen, for a little book reading (a World War II paperback, from the perspective of German infantrymen). Already I'd finished a Karen Kingsbury book that began in Honolulu; "Killing Patton" by Bill O'Reilly; and parts of the Bible and NA basic text book. For the next store run, I started a list of needs and added to it "books." The books provided on the property were limited, and among those, I already read most good ones during prior stays.

1 p.m. Group No. 3 of the day, again on the dining deck. We had to carry all the folding metal and plastic chairs from the classroom up those stairs, including a guy from Big Island who discovered a wooden chair with padding, a King's throne compared with the other chairs that mostly had half-desks. There were some chairs missing a desk, but at least those had padded seats, which I usually claimed for butt relief. As days progressed, so, too, did the back and ass discomfort. Rehab is not really designed for the needs of old folk, another reason to *get rehab right the first time.*

Just this day I learned that some chairs were arranged with the desks set for *left-handed sitters.* Who knew? I also learned from a classmate that "fanny packs are great for shoplifting." Other than learning small lessons, afternoon groups usually suck, especially after fatty lunches in tropical heat. Pre-group small talk is not robust; we're sleepy. The chatter is noticeably lighter when the collective is less caffeinated.

Earlier, I learned that chickens will eat cooked chicken that we toss off the meal deck, and also cooked chicken eggs. You learn a lot in rehabs. After 15 minutes passed and no facilitator, I walked to the office to inform them. The guy who is supposed to be facilitating is on vacation; and no counselors were available to do it. So Herman the PA from the morning got to pinch-hit with a generic "Let's do check-ins!" session. He mentioned that among our group, only one or two would maintain long-term sobriety. I had heard the figure (at least for AA members) was something like 7%; I knew the odds were stacked against us but assumed hardly anyone around me understood the significance. Why burst their bubble, or rain on their parade? A lot of cliches are appropriate, but for me, I was careful not to negatively impact the recovery effort of others with my smarty-pants factoids. Most everyone believed they would *be that person who made it.* The group was supposed to be about "Creating Better Relationships." This would be my fourth one-hour session under this topic, and I still hadn't gotten much from it. The alternative check-ins session was much like the morning. We went around the circle and offered thoughts, feelings, urges, and what we're grateful for. At my turn, I mentioned that today I had the first thoughts of the end this rehab stay. Others offered a wide range of topics, from missing family to getting out of rehab, going to the park upon this session's conclusion, the heat, future housing, the importance of positivity, rooster booby-traps, sober living houses, how you got to this place, and the joy of surviving restriction to use the phone.

2:15 p.m. Kickball. Every Monday at this time we went to a park in a small town nearby. This stay I had yet to play, choosing instead to walk laps, and lightly work out along the way. We hit a mini-market after and I sneakily bought more cans of chew. Maintaining a supply of smokeless tobacco became a top-priority mission.

5 p.m. Dinner. Baked chicken with mashed potatoes.

5:30 p.m. Scheduled was a trip to a weekly event by an organization for men, which is optional. I decline because night gigs cause burn-out especially the older you get. The van leaves and those who stayed back have free time. So we thought.

6:10 p.m. Group No. 4 of the day. Even though it's not listed on the schedule, a PA calls on us remaining on campus to the classroom, to review some rules, namely for bell-ringing after meals (my bad, I'm a nice guy), and rules on how to properly visit the detox nurse. It's our fifth gathering this day, including the morning meditation session.

During evenings without 12-step meetings, I read in my room except 8 to 8:30 p.m. when I visit the main office for medications. There, I take melatonin and typically I'm asleep by 9. Youngsters might stay up until 10, and even wander about outside, but right around "lights out" time they get corralled back to a dorm. That last hour before lights out is usually quiet.

Tuesday, Aug. 6

6 a.m. Woke up with the sound of the usual early morning client scuffling, then walked to the office for hot water for an instant coffee jug. Smoke deck opens at 6, and on this day I had a cigarette to enjoy with the first caffeine. Gave away three cigarettes to a friend in need. Got a second jug of coffee and awaited the 7 a.m. call for meds. Then I wrote until the first group, the short morning meditation weekday sessions. My new young roommate somehow sleeps past the rooster calls outside our window. I'm jealous.

Outside the office, I overheard a relatively new guy lobbying a PA to get moved from our hall to Dorm A, which is more of a cabin than the elongated barracks where we reside. Long before, I was offered to move to Dorm A, but at that moment was quite happy with the crowd we had in Dorm B. In my experience, these types of decisions can be based on choosing the environment with the fewest dumbasses. A lesser-of-two-evils thing. For Dorm A, I found it interesting to see how fast dudes get lured there by a huge living room with a couch, and twice the number of bathrooms, and a wood deck for leisure time. What they don't know is that double the amount of trouble seems to come from A. The past two weeks alone, three guys were "demoted" back to our barracks for various infractions, including constant tardiness, smoking after hours behind a building, or basic juvenile shit. We had a tall, skinny light-black guy missing teeth who was 31 in age but 13 in maturity level, return. For Dorm B inhabitants, it conveyed that our home turf was not a good place; it was *where they sent troublemakers.* Lucky us. (He walked out of the program not long after, and died in 2025 at a big coastal park in Kihei, likely drug-related). As the flunkees returned, I spent more time outside for less noise. Our barrack hallway echoed badly.

I had a decently long chat, on a randomly placed bench, with three of the women. This place is sometimes lax with the gender comingling. They give warnings weekly about the no-no's of over-conversing with the opposite sex, yet … last night before bed I heard at least two male voices among the girls smoking area up on the dining deck. Apparently they were playing a board game up in darkness. The PA who just hours ago lectured us on the topic didn't even leave the office, instead diddling on his mobile phone. Still, four weeks into my stay here, and I'm unaware of any coupling. Typically there's one or two. I always warn other dudes, you *don't go looking for a Cadillac in a junk yard.* Rehabs are the worst place for finding love. Nonetheless, clients still try. Very rarely does it work out long-term.

7:30 a.m. Meditation. Herman once again welcomes us. Usually on Tuesdays and Thursdays we have guided meditation sessions, hosted by staffers or volunteers who do it well. You can almost *feel* that some counselors are new, because *they care.* Long-time counselors can get jaded after years of hearing tons of bullshit. Others might go into Auto Mode, kind of a bureaucratic state where they clock in and out and wait for retirement. I can't fathom how some counselors do it over many years.

Today, it's a new counselor from Iran, a nice guy who kind of got pushed around by clients in a regular group session the week prior. He's very good at leading guided meditation sessions, and I appreciate it. Newcomers will learn in AA (hopefully) that the prayer and meditation combo is the 11th Step. It's included in the steps as another tool to help with recovery maintenance. Mindfulness helps keep you in the moment, in the present, fitting the "One day at a time" mantra. Don't look too far ahead. I find it helps. You don't have to be clean and sober the rest of your life; you just have to be clean and sober *today.*

At the end, client comments as usual ranged broadly. A dude from Dorm A closed with an ode to the rooster who welcomes him from right outside his window at 3 a.m. each morn. I make a mental note.

8 a.m. Breakfast. BIG. Scrambled eggs, sausages, two pancakes. *Way* more than I usually eat. Afterward, the usual, chores which for me means sweeping the dining deck and stairs. After that, third coffee jug. Planning for a long one.

9 a.m. Group No. 1 today, **Co-occurring Disorders**, the first of our two one-hour sessions weekly on the topic. All of us are considered "dual diagnosis," which means we've been designated with more than one mental ailment. I have been diagnosed with substance abuse disorder – like nearly everyone in rehab (except those who don't bother with a medical prognosis). Doctors have also decided that I suffer from major depression and generalized anxiety disorder (GAD). There's a cute little blond from Washington state here. She's smart and funny and I admire her. She couldn't be older than 30, and already with two small children and a meth problem. Another newcomer is who I call Peppermint Patty, a tall, very white-skinned redhead with a crazy stretched-out Afro atop her head and tattoos all over the legs that she did herself. She rarely shuts up. At first to the fellas I called her Pippi Longstalking, but those around me were too young to know about the fictional character with long crazy pigtails. At least some of them knew Peppermint Patty from the "Peanuts" cartoons with Charlie Brown. Today, she sits next to the 31-year-old light-skinned black guy who we suspect has autism. His brother plays in the NFL; yet he is entangled with the legal system in two states. It should be an interesting session.

The director of the whole recovery program (almost universally called Program Director at rehabs) is hosting the group. We're outside on the deck again, and since there's no whiteboard, she made it a simple "process group" session, e.g. she provides a topic, and we share our thoughts about it. First, we kill time with self-introductions plus adding our favorite flower. Don't ask. I said hula flower, the yellow version of the hibiscus that's the Hawaii state flower. Not everyone here knew this.

The director asked, "Talk about challenges you've had in treatment." I started: chronic talking. Why does everyone have to talk so much? Especially *during* group sessions, even when the host speaks and some of us want to hear. We're all together 24-7. What more can we possibly discuss? Is it nerves? A way to be purposely annoying? The director pondered the _why_. Maybe people are not comfortable with silence. The blond from Washington confirmed that yes, she has insecurities. She feels a need for everyone around her to be happy, so the thought is that maybe talking could help others nearby. Then there was discussion about core beliefs, defense mechanisms … a lively discussion. There were what I call Clock-Eaters, who provide over-thought ramblings good for nurturing a feeling that at least the clock is moving, which we all monitor excessively. There are mentions of hyper-vigilance. Peppermint Patty mentioned not trusting people; trust when high on drugs; how to read people; mantras that can fuel addiction. A potpourri of thoughts.

I heard that if you maintain a negative mantra in your head – e.g. "Fuck that guy!" – that's how you'll feel. Halfway through this session, I'm already dreading the next group, the second of three each week where we use a dated workbook. At the end, we're asked to offer one negative core belief, and one positive. Then to do this also for mantras. Nothing memorable surfaces.

10:15 a.m. My Personal Journey, the workbook again. The poor-luck new counselor gets this read-along exercise, just a week after pretty much losing control of a group. I knew the situation was serious because at the session's start the program director sat in, as if to monitor (albeit briefly). But it's a different week in rehab; dynamics always change the feel or mood of us all collectively. It's fascinating to watch for those with interest in sociology, the study of society.

Last week there was drama with the always-tardy guy, plus another client I called Rainman for his ability to talk randomly like the Dustin Hoffman character in the motion picture with Tom Cruise. Rehabs are never the same comparing Day One with the final day. (I also call this client Boomhauer, after the mumbling character in the TV cartoon "King of the Hill," a nickname many other clients will use for the grouchy dude, never to his face of course). When dudes annoy you, veteran rehabbers remind themselves that this is temporary, and that weasels often eject themselves by doing dumb things. People discharge or disappear, dramas come and fade, new people arrive. A circle-of-life thing.

This place now is not what it was two weeks before. Graduates "coin out" with a brief ceremony before leaving, and it seemed like we had a mad rush of them when I started. So a lot of guys who early on supplied me with cigarettes, or who annoyed me, are gone. Some new annoying guys arrived, but overall the place felt less clique-ish. That's a good thing.

Part of the annoyance at this moment is because earlier we had a lot of guys in what is called drug court, and clients who'd been here before. Return customers arrive comfortable, and some in this batch started doing shit like reserving seats at meals. Guys who asked for a lot, like for cigarettes, but rarely said "thank you." At this point in my rehab, money had arrived, so I bought a boatload of tobacco and coffee, and I'd resolved a banking matter so it was easy to shift into cruise control. In previous rehabs, I might have resorted to clock-watching and calendar-checking. This time, I shifted my perception from that of a person "just surviving" rehab, to kind of enjoying this, my (supposed) last rehab. I'd reminisce, remembering programs past, all the lessons, counselors, characters, the works.

New rehabbers won't have this luxury. It's important to focus on a day at a time, or even one hour at a time, if that's what it takes. A lot of newbies fresh from a run will reach a point of sobriety where they have a hard time *not* thinking about using or drinking. It's not just the chemicals. Some of it has to do with little physical things we do all the time. One can go from touching lips all the time from smoking drugs, to not having to do that. Not helping is a system in rehabs which in reality is necessary, but causes its own problems: the early-rehab "restriction" period. Here, the first two weeks mean no phone calls, so for the most part, fixing serious problems with friends, family, or finances gets delayed. You're forced into not thinking about things that you *should* be thinking about. Things like shelter and how you'll eat right after rehab. Mostly, money matters. But remember, that means thinking ahead to the future, and for addicts that's trouble. For true emergencies a counselor could allow brief use of a phone. During the previous rehab stay, my counselor knew my old landlord and let me call to see if I could have a bed in six weeks. That helped eliminate a huge worry: where to live after rehab. I found it very helpful.

Here in this (supposedly) last stay, I had that money anxiety, only to a lesser extent. What I learned from others once I was allowed to use the house phone, is that just prior to coming here, apparently I got loud with my landlord, and she was about to seek a restraining order (before my ex and a friend came and got me out of there). When my brain cleared in detox, I had this thought that, if I completed treatment, I could just return to my old rented room. However, after patiently waiting those first two weeks, I called my ex who said no way would the landlord take me back. This caused a day or so of panic, and mild depression, until I had an opportunity to call the landlord and learn the truth. New rehabbers: *never assume*. Don't believe everyone is pissed at you. Make calls. Verify. Get an opportunity to smooth things out. Don't over-dwell or stew on assumptions.

My landlord already had a solution. She is a survivor of abuse by an alcoholic husband, so I knew there was no chance I'd be allowed to stay there long-term. However, in my mind I knew that I'd at least need time to look for a new place. That was my planned beg when calling my landlord: please allow a little more time. She was ready. My lease was to expire at the end of the following month anyway, and she asked to cut a month off that contract, in exchange for being allowed to remain there the rest of the current month after I discharged. That would be nine days, and since I had a backup plan to stay with Karen temporarily if needed, I took it.

At the end of this group session, some drama, finally. Well, at least for me. The new counselor asked everyone, Why are we always in such a hurry for group to end? As if we had somewhere to go. I started, saying for me it was physical; the hard chairs were unforgiving, and some classes were too long. Someone else said boredom, that some curriculum topics were not all that sexy.

Then, out of nowhere, a dude brought up what I'd said in the first group, about too much talking. He said something like, "I'm new to rehab, so sometimes we talk, to ask questions or discuss." That was followed by general complaints about "know-it-alls," or clients who talk like they're "above the rest of us." Another client chimed in, "Yeah, just because you've been here 12 times before … maybe you're the one missing something." A few "yeahs" by other clients later, the session ended.

A humility shot. Not the first time, either. I was targeted in rehabs prior, just not this … aimed. It dawned on me that I needed humility, that I was getting too comfortable and confident. I'd been teaching groups, criticizing others, making up names for certain clients (e.g. Boomhauer), complaining about elements of this program or curriculum, or otherwise. It was rubbing guys the wrong way. To me, that means I was getting in the way of another person's recovery, which just ain't right. So I adjusted my attitude and approach.

I've said in groups, that everyone who walks in the door has a right to the *opportunity* to experience recovery. Be careful, I'd say, because anything could really knock someone off course. It hit me: I might have nudged a guy out early the previous week. Me and other guys ridiculed him fairly hard about sharing too much in group. The eat-the-elephant-in-one-bite thing. He left after completing just three weeks. I felt bad; it was uncool. Rehab discussions can trigger moments of self-reflection. I've learned to be careful and not overly dwell on it.

1 p.m. Gender Group, with my first counselor, now retired but still hosting groups because he's good at it. First question: Guys who have had time clean, what went wrong? What do you plan to do? Once again I went first: "It took me just a week here to realize I wasn't engaged every day with program. I was in a medical program, with IOP classes online, and meds under the care of a psychiatrist … It wasn't enough. I was taking days off. I realized, *I need to do something every day* to be in contact with sober people. I have a Super Group for my support group, but I rarely use them. Now, on days when I miss a meeting, I need to spend at least an hour a day communicating with sober people."

I need to do something every day to remind myself that I have a serious mental illness, that requires daily treatment. I'm not like normal people. I can't just go to a class reunion, at least without a chaperone. There are just things in life *I can no longer do.*

This was followed by a typical group debate, this time on happiness, a subject that always seems to trigger this particular crowd. Weeks prior, there was an extended discussion about the meaning of life, and someone said, "To be happy." The tall skinny light-skinned black thirtysomething going on 13 said, "Happiness is a byproduct of doing things you like." Rehabbers should expect such deep discussions at least a few times a week. They're always good for killing a half hour or more of a session, and sometimes you might actually learn a bit.

Big Island Brian was also here several times, and other programs several times each, but every time it was just to get "off paper." (*Paper* is a term referring to jail, parole, probation, or other government-ordained legal commands.) "This time feels different. I want to do things I enjoy, like ride motorcycles," he said, providing an incentive to be free of constant oversight in rehabs and by the legal system. He was trying to say he's taking this rehab more seriously. It was not always evident, haha.

After that, a lot more talk about the 12 steps, its literature, and the importance of reading it often. The longer you're clean and sober, the more work is needed, they say.

2:15 p.m. Homework. That's how this 75-minute period is worded on the schedule. It's hardly enforced. For me, it means resting before volleyball. I rip through most homework while in group, and if not, free time at night. I don't watch TV, and am not much for sitting around talking story, as the locals call it. Instead on this day, a staffer drove me to the DMV office up there on the mountain, to file for a replacement ID card. There, they found one document unacceptable, requiring a revisit later. They always do at the DMV on Maui. I expect at least two if not four visits for this task. It's as if the department gets funding for each time the front door opens. Back to Aloha House.

3:30 p.m. Volleyball. I played the whole time. My team lost the first three games, then barely won the last, 26-24. Tired and sore.

5 p.m. Dinner. Fish. Bleh. Not the cooking. Just … no fish or fungi for me. I drowned it with Tabasco sauce.

6 p.m. Cognitive Behavioral Interventions (CBI). Known as CBT due its old name which ended with "therapy." Bleh. A 30-minute video on self; and a handout on setting boundaries. Blah blah. It seems CBT was a hot fad not long before. Seeing it cut back to a single session each week indicates it was not as effective as expected.

7:30 p.m. NA meeting. Attended in our classroom, straightforward. Visiting 12-Steppers are usually involved with what is called Hospitals and Institutions, or H&I panels. It's a way for AA (or NA) members with solid clean time to be of service. I found H&I panels to be solid sources of information and experiences. While just out of the Sally and with the No Nonsense group, I served on H&I panels.

8:30 p.m. Meds. Filled out weekly request forms for visitation the upcoming weekend, a list of items I want during the store run Sunday, and a transportation request to visit my bank in Kihei. The forms are all due by each Wednesday morning. Followed by a little reading, then sleep early.

Wednesday, Aug. 7

6:10 a.m. Woke naturally. Two cups of coffee and a cigarette, then meds at 7 and wait to bell ring by 7:20 a.m.

7:30 a.m. Meditation. We went around the room and all offered our feelings, thoughts, urges, and what we are grateful for this day. I said I was grateful for all my colleague clients here, for helping to nudge in the right direction and keep me focused and on-track. I meant it.

8 a.m. Breakfast. Cheese omelette over rice.

8:20 a.m. Chores. Swept deck, napped briefly to rest for the longest group session of the week which is next.

9 a.m. Culture, or Life Skills. Which one, we never knew in advance. Two hours of a massive information dump on your brain. My big challenge usually seems to be determining how much of it relates to recovery. I had my moments with the host during earlier stays asking that point: What's the relevance? This final AH stay, I promised myself not to hurt his feelings. The adage, "If you don't have anything nice to say, don't say anything" applied. I just focused on trying to survive those 120 minutes each week. At least they moved it to the morning. It was during night hours previously, and it was a challenge to stay awake the second half. Today, pretty much a repeat of two weeks prior, last time he was here. Of the five Wednesdays I'd been here to date, this is only the second time we had the actual host. Mostly they would just cancel any group for that time period which was way cool. Other times, a pinch-hitter would jump in, not really fair considering the scheduled length of the session.

* * *

Right about this time, I noticed that I was beginning to get that "eye on departure" feeling, the *time to coast* phase. Your demeanor or temperament will rollercoaster up and down. For many, at about two weeks remaining, guys hit a wall and care less about the rules and structure. This happened with two guys demoted to our dorm. After a few days of whining, they suddenly "saw the light" and acted kind of happy to be there. I've witnessed this phenomenon multiple times.

It's why, when my emotions kick up, like when I was told my landlord didn't want me back, or the day before when I was attacked verbally by two short-timers, I know to keep my cool and let it pass. My first counselor at AH used to say, and continued to say through this final tour, *"Don't let your emotions dictate your actions."* Reminds me of the old Kinks song "Juke Box Music," with the line, "She lets the songs dictate the way that she feels."

So … I'm just transitioning from a state of total dependence on this facility, to planning my first days out. I'm thinking, I need an ID; to visit the Maui Bus depot to see if my backpack, wallet, and/or mobile phone were turned in; if necessary go buy a new phone; begin organizing to move; look for a new place; check in with my doctor about pre-diabetes mixed with alcohol; re-enroll in my chiropractic program; research AA meetings in Kihei; and re-start my beach-exercise routine.

11 a.m. Nap. Break here for unknown reasons.

11:50 a.m. Lunch. Pizza!

12:15 p.m. Nap.

1 p.m. My Personal Journey. The workbook sesh (again) is scheduled, but on this day a special visit by Waikiki Health to offer free health screenings. I volunteered; no HIV or Hep C for me. No matter how confident you are with infection screenings, doubt and anxiety lingers at least a little. I am not totally confident with fast drug or infection tests.

2:15 p.m. Orientation. My fifth and final required session. Meaning, during this period my last two weeks, I can nap more. Kind of dumb making us attend five sessions but only offer it once a week. You're in orientation pretty much your whole stay. (This changed my following visit, the true Last Rehab, when they reduced the number of these sessions and ultimately didn't even ask for the signed sheet).

3:30 p.m. Volleyball. This session I scribbled my name on the ever-present sign-in sheet, but chose the option to walk the parking lot instead. Walked 36 laps, equaling two miles; 30 push-ups; and 30 leg lifts, about half with a stress band. Good workout. Shower.

5 p.m. Dinner. Some kind of hamburger helper with green beans and salad.

5:45 p.m. Made coffee, rang bell.

6 p.m. Criminal Thinking. Again with my first counselor, who mostly hosted groups the first three days of the week. This session turned into "music appreciation," with each of us choosing a song via YouTube. Songs were supposed to relate to recovery. After an old fart chose "Hell's Bells" by AC/DC (by memory I'm pretty sure it was Brian), I chose "11th Hour" by Rancid – a sober artist, and a song mentioning a girl in addiction. I even selected the video which displayed the lyrics. No one got it, and it made me feel old. It was punk, but dated punk rock. The rest of the session was filled with lame pop or wannabe gangster tunes.

7 p.m. Off-site meeting. Optional, to get vanned to a 12-step meeting, which I decline due to oldmanitis. I'm tired, and last time we didn't return until well after 9. I'm usually passed out cold asleep by then. Burnout is real.

Thursday, Aug. 8

6:05 a.m. Woke naturally, walked to set up coffee mug No. 1, had a cigarette. Then coffee mug No. 2. Guess I was feelin' it this morn.

7:30 a.m. Meditation. I mentioned "rehab fatigue" for the second time here, but for the first time in weeks.

8 a.m. Breakfast. Continental, muffin and yogurt.

8:30 a.m. Meds way later than usual, then a fat dip of chewing tobacco.

9 a.m. Co-Occurring Disorders, session two of two this week. I pay attention as I am dual diagnosed. Plus all the caffeine and nicotine. (Just at this moment realizing that guys who arrived here after me are getting discharged before me. What the?!). However, this session gets cut short by about half, as the program director chose for us to "process" the Lahaina fire disaster exactly a year prior. I still have trouble seeing old photos of Front Street and the Wharf, which were reduced to ashes.

10:15 a.m. Art Therapy. The program director led us as we painted masks.

11:10 a.m. Break. I went to my room to nap and never returned. This is partially because programs insist that we sign attendance sheets before anything else in groups, lest someone leave or somehow miss signing (and they lose reimbursement). Group sign-in sheets are serious shit. Still, all signed, it frees me to sneak off to sleep.

Noon. Lunch. Mega salad. I feel a tooth ache, may have chipped an upper molar.

1 p.m. Gender Group. With the retired counselor again, the whole session on the 12 steps and sponsors. *Where is gender here?* I thought. Sometimes, group facilitators go cruise control, or choose topics they feel really matter. In this case, the 12 steps seems better for us than gender studies.

2:15 p.m. ECC group. Just for people who need help from a staffer there named Ivan, to do things like get an ID. I think the name has something to do with *extra* something or other. I never remembered. We had good sessions in the past, namely one on credit scores and everything involved with them. This session they asked, "Am I a Good Friend?" Ooh, I'd say to myself. *Deep.*

3:30 to 4:15 p.m. Volleyball. Played. We were well ahead in Game 3, with the teams tied a game apiece, when two women got into a shouting match that wouldn't end, and the staffers playing had to intervene, ending our match. It was the first raised voices I'd heard here, several weeks into program. At the following meal time, three staffers stood around the women's dining platform (separate from the one connected to the kitchen for men; poor gals had to carry meals and drinks through a winding route to sit and eat, all in the name of keeping us separated). Staff anticipated lingering animosity between the screamers, which did not materialize.

5 p.m. Dinner. Roast with veggies. Ran out of salad. Big break afterward, before a final two-hour group, kind of tough at the end of four full days of grouping.

6 p.m. Culture Group. As if Wednesday morning's two-hour marathon wasn't enough. This counselor, an older lady with a funky woke haircut who came from working at a homeless program, chose to play the movie "Grand

Torino." Oh well, I'm expecting my counselor to come pull me from group any time, for our weekly meeting, which seems to occur later each week, not unusual at rehabs. She never came. I bet our weekly sit-downs will end up on Friday afternoons. Then what? Return to Mondays? Haha.

8 p.m. Meds. Night means eye drops for glaucoma, and melatonin for sleep.

8:30 p.m. Counselor sends someone to my room to call me out to visit. We sat outside on a nearby sloped grass, with a new, more *seasoned* gal (read: younger than me but not close to age 23), where we all talked about a huge Cheshire moon, and how my counselor always promised to meet. Haha! My counselor then said we'll meet tomorrow (Friday, told ya), 1 to 2 p.m. (For the record, Friday is a packed schedule; hardly a break to be found there).

9 p.m. Bed. Out fast, exhausted.

Friday, Aug. 9

6:10 a.m. Woke naturally to the first voices outside the room.

7 a.m. Meds. Coffee, then kept reading a book about German army infantry all-stars. I'm not making this up, that's what the book called them, "all-stars."

7:20 a.m. Rang bell.

7:30 a.m. Meditation. With Isaiah the cool PA with the big motorcycle, limp from a biking accident, and ZZ Top goatee. Looks like his first time facilitating. He's smiling big, which is rather rare in the morning although Herman does a good job. Isaiah promises a fast one. There's a lot of whining, and rumors that they are short on staff due to some holiday so we might not go to the beach this day. Isaiah: "I am thankful for this job and being here with you." Amen. We go around the room and say our thoughts, what we're grateful for, etc. A client here just received a letter from his insurance provider stating they will only cover 14 days. Sound familiar? The always-tardy guy is leaving in six days, and another, who I helped with an essay required for drug court, to be gone in four. The King of the Kitchen Mafia, who I'm having Rooster Wars with, lectures us on the history of AA. Isaiah mentioned how neat it is to start each day with gratefulness. Reminds me of when I first started attempting recovery in 2009, at 6:15 a.m. almost every day. It was a good way to do it, in my experience. Awaken, skip a shower and just slip on shoes or slippahs, shorts and a tee, and go. Free coffee! The broken molar now is causing a little face pain. My oldmanitis woes never cease.

8 a.m. Breakfast. Absolute bomb portions of scrambled eggs and sausage.

9 to 11:30 a.m. Beach. Two vans take us all to Kanaha Beach in the northeast side of Kahului. Often this beach is wind-blown, but this early we enjoy time in the water. I read and sunbathed, and then played two games of volleyball on a sand court. Nicknamed one always-falling gal Pigpen. I think Peppermint Patty played, too.

Noon. Lunch. Sloppy Joe sandwiches.

1 p.m. Can't remember the group topic. The counselor pulled me out as promised. In her office, we went over past writing assignments, which I always completed on time. I asked a few questions and was assigned more homework.

2 p.m. Community Meeting. A weekly opportunity for staff to provide program or facility updates, and for us to provide feedback. Staff went over major rules, and then we were allowed to bring up issues. All three court-ordered clients whined; two about having to do 45 days when some have to do "just" 30; another about getting three write-ups in a 24-hour period. In the end? We all agreed he could leave at any time. (Which Write-Up King did shortly after; he died rehab-free and homeless in 2025).

3:30 p.m. Anger Management. A weekly end-of-week, long group session where I always said walking in, *"Anger management class pisses me off."* Bad scheduling. My counselor gets the unfortunate assignment of killing a full 90 minutes with this topic, and she's not the most seasoned group presenter so these tend to drag. We coined out one of the Dylans. I noted in my mind that part of the Kitchen Mafia leaves Monday. (At the break, I filled a big coffee mug). Then we watched an episode of "The Office" where Andy punches a hole in a wall and is forced to attend anger management classes. I feel for him, having done about 50 anger management classes during a two-year period thanks to violating restraining orders from Karen. Lesson learned. Near the end, the 31-year-old going on 13 leaves. He had drawn on a desk his name, attached to a glass drug pipe. He had been annoying many by making juvenile mouth noises in groups. He played the victim here, and pouted out the door. Few cared. Rehabs are kind of like early episodes of the TV show "Survivor." People get offed and few care, except people who are relieved that annoying fuckers are gone.

5 p.m. Dinner. Cooked tuna pasta with salad. Right after, free night, no groups, no night meetings. Hallelujah.

8 p.m. Meds. Out by 9. Us older clients really start to feel it at the end of a series of packed weekdays.

WEEKEND

Saturday, Aug. 10

6:10 a.m. Wake to the noise of a very loud voice down the hall seemingly talking loudly to himself, or to a door, or piece of furniture. No one else is talking. This goes on for a while. Before I go get coffee, I walk down the hall to comfort Loud Man's roommate. "Gary," I say as nicely as possible, "We're so sorry." Then I go back to my room, shut the door, sip coffee, and continue reading Nellie Bowles' latest book. It's superb. I bought it at the start of summer and was deep into it, then relapsed and lost it like I lose everything in relapse. To my glee, I saw it sitting atop the main office lobby fridge, and waited a few days before grabbing it. Stoked. A side note: when I made the comment to Gary, his roommate, the loud self-talker, was Brian of Big Island. I said it outside the door without showing my face. My roommate at the time happened to be walking down the hall and told me Brian said, "Who was that? Is that Gump?" A joke between us because he always sat on this lone bench in the center of campus like Forest Gump at his bus stop, and I'd yell "Forrest Gump!" and point when walking by. Then he started yelling "Gump!" at me randomly. Despite the Loud Man annoyance, Brian and I had some hearty laughs. He's a big old grouchy Big Islander who's only here by court order. Somehow I got along with him. He laughs off my sarcasm, and says some of the funniest shit in group. This morning, a whole bunch of people addicted to the sound of their own voice caucused at the bench. They'll talk a lot about nothing until the meal bell rings.

8 a.m. Breakfast. Continental, got a chocolate-chip muffin and blueberry yogurt. Keeping breakfast light. (Eventually I would actually lose weight compared with when I walked in).

8:15 a.m. Meds.

8:30 a.m. Double Scrub. I got assigned to spray off and clean the whole men's smoking deck (which also serves as the lady's meal-eating area). Then, on my own because I was bored, I grabbed a long hose and sprayed chicken poo off sidewalks.

10 a.m. Expectations. This is the only group scheduled for the day. It is rarely fulfilling. Then … sheer boredom. It's only a half-hour class, and I still never understood why it was necessary. Maybe a safety valve, in case someone did something dumb on Friday night and staff reserved the time in case they needed to bitch at us. I heard someone say we were out of laundry detergent, which reminded me of something the program director had mentioned, that the organization was at the end of its fiscal year so funds were limited. At least I was here when they got the air-conditioning in the classroom – a $15,000 project and reminder that I was not at TTC or the Sally.

10:15 a.m. Nap and read.

Noon. Lunch. Reheated frozen shrimp over buttered noodles. Blech.

12:20 p.m. I did chores on my own, napped, and read. Eventually I chose to hand-wash two light athletic shirts good for keeping cool at volleyball, preparing to get into the following week without having to do a laundry load, anticipating a few days for them to get laundry detergent. Rehab All-Stars know to think ahead.

3:15 p.m. Sat at Gump bench, writing this book, in case visitors arrive. By this time I just submitted a visitors request form listing anyone who *might* visit each weekend. I'm not a fan of telephone calls and wasn't about to call people on Friday to pressure anyone to come. I always told them they could if they wanted, but it was not required. After the 3:30 p.m. visit starting time passed, I walked to my room to nap.

3:50 p.m. Visitation. Karen arrives, late as usual, an ongoing joke. Fun talk, caught up on all the work on her properties, and we discussed logistics for my discharge Aug. 22. Officially Aug. 21 is my last day of groups. I'm free at 6 a.m. the day after. That's when real life returns. She leaves at 4:30.

5 p.m. Dinner. Stew over rice, with salad.

5:20 p.m. Chores, read, nap. Don't leave room for a while.

8:05 p.m. Meds. Then out asleep even without melatonin. Thoughts about exactly which meds I might drop. I take way too many pills daily.

Sunday, Aug. 11

7:20 a.m. No meditation session weekends. Woke to many voices outside my room. A *lot* of new guys, more war stories, a lot of swear words. I feel it's time to go.

7:30 a.m. Meds. For some reason, my health care provider is giving grief, about a co-pay to refill a single med. Just another thing for me to look into, or worry about. It's amazing just how big American bureaucracy has become, public or private. I abhor bureaucracy.

8 a.m. Breakfast. Scrambled eggs and baked Vienna sausages.

9:15 a.m. Store Run. Vanned to Kahului, to shop first at a little market for tobacco, then to Walmart. Spent $107, got two T-shirts, new slippahs, peanuts (rooster food), real coffee for everyone (staff provided a machine in the office lobby, but we had to provide the coffee; after weeks of nothing I decided to treat the house). I bought smokes for my roommate and a young friend who eventually moved to Georgia; skin lotion; shaving cream; aloe lotion; stevia leaf extract sweetener; etc. I'm a lucky one here having money to spend, so I usually buy stuff for others to repay for the generosity I received when I arrived.

Noon. Lunch. Fried chicken patty sandwiches, baked beans, and corn.

1 p.m. Transition Skills. With the pretty new counselor. It's the only group on Sunday. This one's about defense mechanisms. I'm too tired to participate. Another 90-minute group. Rehabs have not caught on to the fact that the attention spans of Americans are now measured in seconds, not hours or even minutes. The group slowly got a little better. We broke into groups of two, and me and Tardy Guy did a brief acting skit where I asked him four questions about excuses to do drugs too much, and he rationalized ad lib through it all. Hilarious. There are certain phrases, or actions, or even postures, that most addicts use. Tardy Guy nailed the excuses to a T, a reason most of us found it really funny. The counselor just gave a curious look.

2:30 to 5 p.m. Nap. Skipped for the first time a church they set up in the classroom at 4 p.m. each Sunday. It's a very good worship service by a band of players who survived addiction and incarceration, with a sermon by a pastor from the Kihei ministry of the huge King's Cathedral Church. I'd attended each since it started, but on this day I felt fatigued.

5 p.m. Dinner. Beef stroganoff. Good. Then chores, and reading. Now into a Grisham book I found.

8 p.m. Meds. Took 3 mg of melatonin. Still had a hard time falling asleep. It was hot, and our room still did not have a fan, since mine was stolen by Day 3. It rained lightly overnight, and got humid. Asleep by 9:30 p.m. – the end of the fifth of the 6-week program.

CHAPTER 9

ALOHA HOUSE NO. 4, 2025

The Long and Winding Road

After completing Aloha House No. 3 in late August 2024, because this book was mostly written out in draft form by that point, I threw a serious-sized wrench into the endeavor. I relapsed immediately. How was I supposed to now write and pitch a book related to recovery? The answer is, *this is not a book about recovery*. This tome is about rehabs, facilities offering housing, education, and other services. It's merely my observations and opinions about programs I participated in, with details and some background to provide contrast between rehabs. Some details, such as segments in between rehab stays, or the chapter about 2017, are to convey how hard life can be trying to live with untreated addiction. Maybe there's a book on recovery to come, who knows? I'm leaning toward a follow-up to this book, tentatively to be titled, "Sober Living House All-Stars." Plenty to work with there.

In terms of recovery, I got lucky, and honestly still feel blessed to be alive. With the help of the same woman who brought me to Maui, along with lifelong friend James Swanson, I was able to snap out of the final relapse quickly. I lucked upon the very same bed in the very same sober living house, thanks to the forgiving angels who run that program, where I spent the rest of the year transcribing and organizing this book.

I don't have answers to help someone get clean or sober. I have not attained lasting sobriety, so I don't know what it takes. All I can offer are observations, and things I think *might help*, as well as a lot of warnings about things that can *hurt*. Since every human being has a brain unique to each self, recovery differs by individual. Like my very first treatment physician said early, addiction is a combination of many factors, among them biology, heredity, and social circumstances. Each of us starts with our own brain, which gets molded by experiences, which makes us all even more individualistic.

It's a reason why some people can attend one or a few rehabs and get it and remain clean for years, like my friend Molly from AIA No. 1. Hers may have depended more on the societal element – she was young and very much loved her mother, who she really wanted to make happy. Although I had three kids, they all were in their teens and luckily very self-sufficient, and when the wife left and landed a job to support them, no one depended on me or my recovery. Different situations. Not to use Molly and I as pure examples of this phenomenon, but another thing that made our challenges different is, she started young, and while she had plenty of horrible moments in addiction, they weren't stretched out over many years. I would imagine that snapping out of it in detox, then getting information to help deal with the past, could be easier when horrible memories aren't piled up. I didn't start trying until I'd been in the partying game 25 years – so I had a mountain of bad memories to get past. I had a quarter-century of physical abuse and mental anguish to work through. All that said, Molly's achievement is miraculous, and I can't love her enough for what she did for her mother, and later, her daughters. Truly heartwarming.

Yet, for every Molly and one-rehab wonders, there are lost souls like myself who keep punishing themselves repeatedly. In rehabs, staffers probably will say something like, you didn't create your addiction in a day, so don't expect to recover that quickly. We all worked long and hard to maintain our addiction. We expended a tremendous amount of energy and sucked up a lot of time keeping it going. If we could only dedicate that same level of energy and attention to *stopping* use of alcohol or drugs, imagine what could get accomplished. It's a reminder, often repeated, because addicts very easily and quickly forget just how bad and unmanageable their lives had become.

* * *

So how did I do it? Well, let's begin with the fact that *I still haven't done it*. To reach a state of lucidity to write all this, I had a sort-of cosmic realization in which the addiction just seemed to *leave*. It wasn't immediate, and cannot be linked to any program or particular tool or tactic. It's just that once my brain again cleared and I found my life again packed into a house with a bunch of guys, a sense of relief came. Sure, I returned to the psychiatrist and the meds, but besides the sober living house rules, and a lot of medical appointments playing catch-up, I didn't do much else. I didn't do what I promised to get totally engaged with AA. I attended a single meeting early on, mainly to help a friend in her own recovery, and rarely returned. I did in fact find an online weekly SMART Recovery meeting, and revisited a melded AA-Bible meeting nearby, and try to make those consistently. It's not that AA does not work; it works for millions of alcoholics globally. It's just that over many years engaged with the program, it felt like it just wouldn't work *for me*. Additionally, and this can be important for some, I found that constantly hearing and talking about drinking made me thirsty.

I found the biggest key is *acceptance*. The AA big book conveys this clearly. For myself, it was a matter of accepting that I have a serious mental illness; that I cannot do many things non-addicted people can; and that if I don't dedicate the utmost seriousness to this malady, it will maim or even kill me. In the end, the horror and feeling of helplessness during that final week of drinking burned images in my brain of what was to come if the drinking continued – none of it good. I wished to avoid it. It may sound silly, as if I simply just got sick of it all, but somehow my brain relaxed, accepted, adapted, and began healing. I became much more at ease. Thanks partially to a lot of lessons learned along the way, including in AA, things that used to cause anxiety now do not. I finally discovered how to live life on life's terms – not on my terms. Much involves focusing on *not trying to control everything*. Shit happens in life. We have no power over it, no matter how hard we try. I can't control being born with a birth defect, or with a mental illness maybe passed genetically. We can't control bad luck like car accidents, nor can we control how other people influence our feelings, like hostile bosses. People will always either bring us joy and contentment, or they will piss us off.

The main thing is *learning how to handle it*. I think recovery is less about fighting a particular chemical, and more about being able to cope with life and challenges it presents, situations that push to the poisons. Some people are born with that skill, others get it fairly young, and others like me have to work like hell to get it.

To the potential new rehabber I would say: What do you have to lose by trying rehab? Ask yourself, *Why am I even thinking about it?* Hopefully that presents a goal, like the ability to enjoy watching a ballgame without getting smashed, to work toward. Is that goal important to you? Is it important for the people around you? Do you care about those close to you, family members and friends who love you?

* * *

Aloha House No. 4 lasted from early May to June 23, 2025. I had a new counselor, and she was wonderful. She set up a cake-and-ice cream party for my birthday June 10 – my first birthday party in at least two decades. I mentioned that I'd done every holiday in rehabs over the years, like Independence Day, Christmas, etc., but never my birthday. My counselor noted this, then delivered.

Something really different happened in this rehab, and mainly it was because of all the writing about past rehab experiences. My attitude went right into Humility Mode. No more know-it-all statements, no practical jokes. I spoke when asked, or if I really had information to share that might help someone. I spoke much less, and discovered that *it actually helped*, in fact a lot. I shut up and listened. The way it should have been all along.

I already had an apartment paid for in advance, and besides some medical matters my counselor hustled with, I had few concerns out in the real world. Karen was still around to help, and visited more than once, but overall my plate was cleared to do nothing but focus on program.

At this "final" rehab, very early I was informed that I might have damage or problems with my cerebellum, causing dizziness and loss of balance, especially when I added alcohol. Herman drove me to urgent care, because I was having difficulty walking, especially in detox but also lingering into residential. Something was off, and the detox nurse suggested a physician's opinion. I was told by someone (a detox nurse or client) that it seemed like a thyroid issue, which is what I told the urgent care doc immediately. He just as quickly dismissed it, and suspected cerebellum issues. He recommended an MRI and consultation with a neurologist. After rehab, the neurologist found nothing urgently serious, but noticed a reduced volume in the brain, something to do with the very ends of arteries. I was prescribed a pill to prevent a heart attack or stroke due to concern about cholesterol with these tiny, apparently shrinking artery tips.

So, I started the final rehab with belief that I might have brain damage. Talk about humbling. It kept me pretty quiet for a week or two, but eventually the demands of the program forced my worries aside and I felt many times a supreme gratefulness, that I would get the help I needed. Not just for recovery, but also for physical ailments, some of which may have been exacerbated by drinking. Previously diagnosed was glaucoma, scoliosis, and arthritis all over, severe neck arthritis is why I was approved for federal disability payments. Oldmanitis was hitting hard, and it won't get better especially if I drink. I very well might not have another recovery left in me. The very next drink could permanently maim, or even kill. The concept of wet brain scares me. I've met wet brain victims, and it's alarming.

This rehab, I learned quite a bit, and much credit belongs with staff at Aloha House. Much appreciation to: my first counselor, Nic, whose advice on program (and the importance of physical fitness for recovery, as well as to combat oldmanitis) was invaluable; Herman the PA for his morning sermons and friendly chats; Cassidy and Sarah, my last (and quite patient) counselors; PAs like Kawena, Nara, Mia, Sam, Bob, Jeannie, Elisha, Josiah, Rob, and others who were always so nice; guys like Ivan who always seemed spot-on speaking; and Sheryl the firm yet fair intake angel who always found a way to get me a detox bed quickly. When any of these folks spoke, I listened, and urged other patients to do the same.

My colleagues were cool and there was little riff-raff. At one point, some asshole brought in meth and took out five clients, and it caused a stir, but the program handled it well. Once again, somehow Aloha House was even better than before, and we're talking in just the year I was away. I spent many moments walking around shaking my head, wondering how they did it. Why can't all rehabs do the same and adjust to improve? It's not like Aloha House was forced to get better. Heck, it could be said it had little competition and the need to expend money and energy to improve is not there. But they seemed to make adjustments with each visit.

Besides the meth incident, the only recurring drama seemed to involve vapes, those little nicotine-vapor gizmos, that everyone seemed to be sneaking in (and getting caught with). Hearing about the vapes from staff consumed hours of my time there cumulatively. I still don't know why vapes are banned, and said so in all-client meetings with staff present. I understand they could be fiddled with to fill with dope, but how often does that actually happen? Is it worth all the time and energy expended to discuss all the time, and to constantly conduct searches? I can assume that many other rehabs also ban vapes and vaping. Like it was featured in *Rehab Today* magazine or something, as I like to say.

I don't vape so besides all the lost time, it wasn't an issue for me. I do, however, chew tobacco, and Aloha House banned it in 2021, forcing me to smoke cigarettes. Therein lies why I question the vape matter (as well as the chew ban). Nothing is worse for your health in terms of tobacco use than smoking cigarettes. Nothing. I hate smoking, yet in two rehab facilities felt I *had to*, because I couldn't chew. (Ultimately, usually, I'd somehow buy chew and then go out of my way to hide it; I admit it, one of my few big rehab shenanigans).

Minor issues compared with program, and in AH No. 4, it was maybe the best program yet. Kudos to Aloha House.

I coined out in late June and, just like the year prior, did nothing I promised post-program, except attend an AA meeting the same afternoon as discharge. After that, nothing, and I admit, I relapsed. So, I made a dramatic change and left my private apartment, for the old sober living house I'd lived in mostly since 2021. Aloha House warned me of their concerns that I would leave program for the apartment, and not get in a structured situation like a sober living house program. They were right, and by late-July 2025 I was back in a CARM house, where Karen and James Swanson said I always seemed to do well. I write these final words from a kitchen island on Molokai Hema Street, safe and sound with hopes to keep helping addicts in need.

Mahalo to everyone for all the care, love, and attention. This addict needs it. I hope to spend the rest of my life trying to help others avoid becoming a Rehab All-Star.

CHAPTER 10

LESSONS LEARNED

Looking back at all my rehabs, there seems to be two types of lessons learned: micro and macro. Micro lessons are little tools and tactics that help along the way in rehabs or very early recovery, things like how to meditate, or identify triggers. Rehabbers will absorb many micro lessons, most helpful, some not so much. The macro lessons are broad, and if applied can bring noticeable progress. Here are macro lessons I feel I learned at each stop.

- **AIA Nos. 1 to 3.** Be grateful, and humble. You don't know all; that's why you're there.
- **Salvation Army Nos. 1 and 2.** Don't waste time; grab the reins for your life for yourself and take actions to move forward; understand humility, because life always could be worse; and be patient.
- **TTC Nos. 1 and 2.** Be patient, avoid bad attitudes, and remain in gratefulness always. (Notice trends so far?)
- **Redgate Nos. 1 and 2.** Make recovery the No. 1 priority in your life. Be grateful for little things, like the opportunity to laugh along with colleagues.
- **Aloha House Nos. 1 to 4.** Healthy routines evolve into helpful habits. Don't underestimate the value of spirituality, any way you can attain it, in recovery. It may be right before your eyes. Have patience and keep the faith.

SPECIAL THANKS

This book wouldn't exist if not for the rehab facilities and personnel that did their best to try to provide a foundation to work from toward my personal pursuit of long-term, lasting sobriety. Regardless of criticisms, and I admit there were plenty, I am happy they exist (or existed). We need more substance abuse treatment centers.

Many thanks to Kristi Earley, Kris Bowen Carrese, Diana Meng, Jackie and Brian Lussky, Jill Dolan, Todd Orozco, Sean De La Cruz, Lena and Jeff Johnson, John Rimmer, Tim Mott, Mike Edwards, Gina and Matt Gooding, Cheeky Palomarez, John Whiteley, Steve Silkin, Marc Weinstein, Michelle Barrelier, Gabriel Garcia, Scott Cleaveland, Jammy Hsu of Taiwan, Brad Chandler, David and Kim Milstien, Pninit Kat, Janelle Falaschi, Raquel Wirth, Paul Webb, and Nicole Blizzard (RIP) – these folks went above and beyond trying to help, or were soothing or trusted confidantes. No one did more or tried harder than Lisa Ridgway Jajko, and I love her for that (along with many other reasons).

For the book, super special thanks to James Swanson, Brittany Harris, Zachary Hyatt, Molly Kennedy, Robin Baty, Karen Smart, and a bunch of former rehab colleagues, including but not limited to Richard Calmet, Josh Caylor, and many others who are in this book but under pseudonyms. Your contributions will never be forgotten.

For my recovery efforts over the years, heartfelt appreciation for the love and attention from Glen Becerra, Steve Sojka, Jim Johnston, Mike Jacob, Mark Benner, Doug and Cheri Burnside, Dan Rosen – these folks went above and beyond trying to help. Much appreciation to Dixie and Scott and the whole team at COA – long live your extraordinary service for those in need in Long Beach! Thank you to Denise Haggerty Novelli, my first success with helping another person get sober – and she's still sober many years later!

Many others provided kindness behind the scenes, like Brooke

Kauffman, my angelic cousin who once somehow tracked me down to get a nurse to stick a wireless ER phone into my ear. (She opened with, "What the fuck are you doing?" Haha! What a miracle). You all know who you are, and I apologize if I can't immediately remember everyone. But know that in my heart, my appreciation for you is full and sincere.

Thank you to all my sponsors, and many people in rehabs, emergency rooms, hospitals, ambulances, psyche wards, sober living houses, AA meetings, 12-step groups, food pantries, soup kitchens, food and clothing banks, courtrooms, and jails. This includes judges, peace officers, and probation officers. Hundreds of people who care. Thank you to all the unnamed street survivors who provided wise words or comfort along the way. I needed it all.

Finally, profound feelings of appreciation for my parents, Ted and Kathy Jajko, who passed away during this process but whose never-ceasing love and care provided inspiration, and incentive to break the cycle of alcoholism in our family. God bless.